FIT AND FUELED

The Ultimate Guide to Nutrition and Exercise for Lasting Weight Loss

— SAMUEL SALAM —

Table of Contents

Introduction:

Fit & Fueled – Your Path to Lasting Weight Loss

Welcome! I'm thrilled you've taken the first step in transforming your life with *Fit & Fueled: The Ultimate Guide to Nutrition and Exercise for Lasting Weight Loss*. After years of dedicated research, many experts in this field have found that there is an understanding of the intricate balance between nutrition and exercise. I can confidently tell you that achieving lasting weight loss is not about quick fixes or unsustainable diets. It's about fueling your body and mind in a way that supports your goals, enhances your energy, and empowers you to live your best life.

In this guide, we'll explore why being fit and fueled is key to lasting weight loss. You'll discover how nutrition and exercise are not opposing forces but complementary tools that, when combined strategically, can unlock your potential for a stronger, healthier, and happier you.

Why Being Fit and Fueled is Key to Lasting Weight Loss

Weight loss is often seen as a battle against the scale, but I'm here to shift your perspective. This journey is about gaining energy, confidence, and control over your health. When you focus on fueling your body with nutritious foods and strengthening it through regular exercise, weight loss becomes a byproduct of a balanced, sustainable lifestyle.

Being *fit* means more than physical strength; it's about resilience, endurance, and vitality. Being *fueled* means providing your body with the right nutrients in the right amounts to power through your day and achieve your fitness goals. Together, these principles create a foundation for weight loss that's not only effective but lasting.

The Balance Between Nutrition and Exercise

One of the biggest myths about weight loss is that it's all about cutting calories or spending hours at the gym. In reality, it's the balance between nutrition and exercise that truly makes a difference. What you eat fuels how you move, and how you move impacts how your body processes and utilizes that fuel.

In this guide, I'll show you how to create this balance for yourself. You'll learn to nourish your body with nutrient-dense foods, including tips for meal prepping and portion control, and how to create a fitness routine that works with your lifestyle, not against it. Whether you're just starting your journey or looking to break through a plateau, this balance is the secret to unlocking lasting success.

How to Use This Guide for Your Personal Transformation

Fit & Fueled is more than just a guide—it's your roadmap to personal transformation. Each chapter is packed with actionable steps, evidence-based strategies, and motivational insights designed to meet you where you are and guide you toward where you want to be.

Start by setting your goals and defining your "why"—your personal motivation for embarking on this journey. From there, explore the chapters on nutrition and exercise, which will provide you with the tools to build a lifestyle that supports lasting weight loss. Finally, use the mindset and habit-forming strategies to overcome challenges and ensure your success for years to come.

This isn't just about losing weight; it's about gaining a new perspective on health and happiness. So, are you ready to take the first step toward a stronger, more energized, and confident you? Let's begin your journey to being truly fit and fueled!

Part 1:
Nutrition for Lasting Weight Loss

Chapter 1

The Power of Eating Smart

Understanding Nutrition Basics: Calories, Macronutrients, and Micronutrients

Nutrition is the foundation of good health, weight management, and fitness. However, it can often seem complicated with the abundance of information available. To make informed choices about what you eat, it's essential to understand the basics of nutrition, particularly the roles of calories, macronutrients, and micronutrients. By grasping these core principles, you can better fuel your body, maintain energy levels, and support your long-term health.

Calories: The Energy Your Body Needs

At its most basic level, a calorie is a unit of energy. Everything you eat and drink contains calories, and your body uses them to perform various functions—from keeping your heart beating to powering physical activities like walking or exercising. Calories are essential for survival, but understanding how many you consume versus how many you burn is key to managing weight.

When you consume more calories than your body uses, the excess is stored as fat, leading to weight gain over time. Conversely, when you consume fewer calories than your body needs, it turns to stored fat for energy, resulting in weight loss. While it's important to monitor calorie intake, not all calories are created equal. The source of these calories—whether they come from proteins, fats, or carbohydrates—matters greatly in how your body uses them.

Macronutrients: The Building Blocks of Nutrition

Macronutrients, often referred to as "macros," are nutrients that provide energy and are needed in large amounts by the body. There are three main macronutrients: proteins, carbohydrates, and Fats. Each plays a unique role in your body's health and functioning.

- **Proteins**: Protein is crucial for building and repairing tissues, especially muscles. It also plays a role in producing enzymes and hormones that regulate bodily processes. Good sources of protein include lean meats, fish, eggs, beans, and plant-based alternatives like tofu or lentils. Protein is also beneficial for weight management because it helps you feel fuller for longer, reducing overeating.
- **Carbohydrates**: Carbohydrates are the body's primary energy source, particularly for brain function and high-intensity physical activities. They come in two forms: simple and complex. Simple carbs, found in sugary snacks and processed foods, provide quick energy but often lead to spikes and crashes in blood sugar levels. Complex carbs, found in whole grains, vegetables, and legumes, provide more sustained energy and are rich in fiber, which aids digestion. For lasting energy and better health, focus on incorporating more complex carbs into your diet.
- **Fats**: Despite their bad reputation, fats are essential for your body. They support cell function, protect organs, and help absorb certain vitamins. However, it's important to choose the right types of fats. Unsaturated fats, found in foods like avocados, nuts, seeds, and olive oil, are heart-healthy and beneficial for overall wellness. Saturated and Trans fats, often found in fried foods and processed snacks, should be limited, as they can contribute to heart disease and other health issues.

Each macronutrient plays a vital role in a balanced diet. For optimal health and weight management, a diet with a healthy balance of protein, carbohydrates, and fats is essential.

Micronutrients: Small But Mighty

Micronutrients are vitamins and minerals that your body requires in smaller amounts compared to macronutrients, but they are equally important. They do not provide calories or energy, but they support critical functions such as immune system strength, bone health, and energy production.

- **Vitamins**: These are organic compounds that support various bodily functions. For instance, Vitamin C is crucial for immune function, while Vitamin D supports bone health by aiding in calcium absorption. Most vitamins must come from food sources because the body cannot produce them in sufficient quantities.
- **Minerals**: These include elements like calcium, potassium, and iron, which are essential for processes like muscle contraction, nerve function, and oxygen transport. Iron, for example, is a key component of hemoglobin, which carries oxygen in the blood, while calcium is vital for strong bones and teeth.

A diet rich in fruits, vegetables, whole grains, and lean proteins provides the necessary vitamins and minerals for optimal health. Deficiencies in micronutrients can lead to various health problems, so it's important to consume a diverse, nutrient-dense diet.

Common Myths About Dieting and Weight Loss

In the quest for weight loss, there is no shortage of advice—much of which can be confusing or downright misleading. With so much information out there, it's easy to fall prey to common myths that promise quick fixes or radical transformations. However, understanding the truth behind these myths is essential for making informed decisions and achieving long-term success. Let's debunk some of the most common dieting and weight loss myths.

Myth 1: Carbs Make You Gain Weight

One of the most persistent myths is that all carbohydrates cause weight gain. While low-carb diets can be effective for some, the idea that carbs are inherently bad is false. Carbohydrates are a primary source of energy, particularly for high-intensity physical activities and brain function. The key is to focus on the type and quantity of carbs you consume.

Simple carbohydrates, such as sugary snacks, white bread, and processed foods, can lead to spikes in blood sugar, which may contribute to weight gain. However, complex carbohydrates, like whole grains, vegetables, and legumes, provide sustained energy and are packed with fiber, which helps regulate digestion and keeps you full longer. Instead of cutting out carbs entirely, opt for healthier, whole food sources that provide nutrients and fuel your body effectively.

Myth 2: Skipping Meals Helps You Lose Weight

Many people believe that skipping meals, especially breakfast, will help them cut calories and lose weight faster. However, skipping meals can have the opposite effect. When you skip meals, your body may enter a state of hunger, causing you to overeat later in the day. It can also slow down your metabolism, as your body attempts to conserve energy due to a lack of consistent fuel.

Additionally, skipping meals may lead to poor food choices when hunger strikes. You're more likely to grab quick, unhealthy snacks when your blood sugar is low. Instead of skipping meals, focus on eating balanced, nutrient-dense meals throughout the day to maintain your energy levels and support steady metabolism.

Myth 3: Eating Fat Makes You Fat

The idea that eating fat leads directly to body fat is another widespread myth. While it's true that fats are more calorie-dense than proteins or carbohydrates, fats are essential for overall health and can actually aid in weight loss when consumed in moderation. Healthy fats, such as those found in avocados, nuts, seeds, and olive oil, support important bodily functions, including hormone regulation and the absorption of fat-soluble vitamins.

Incorporating healthy fats into your diet can also help you feel fuller for longer, reducing cravings and overeating. The key is to avoid unhealthy fats, such as trans fats and excessive amounts of saturated fats, which are linked to heart disease and weight gain.

Myth 4: You Have to Do Intense Workouts Every Day to Lose Weight

Another common myth is that weight loss requires grueling, daily workouts. While regular exercise is important for overall health and weight management, you don't need to engage in extreme workouts every day to see results. Overtraining can actually be counterproductive, leading to injury, burnout, or exhaustion.

The most effective exercise routine is one that you can sustain long-term. This can include a mix of cardio, strength training, and flexibility exercises. Consistency is more important than intensity. Even moderate-intensity activities like walking, swimming, or yoga can contribute significantly to weight loss when combined with proper nutrition.

Myth 5: Quick-Fix Diets and Detoxes Are Effective for Long-Term Weight Loss

Quick-fix diets, detoxes, and cleanses often promise rapid weight loss, but they rarely deliver lasting results. Many of these diets involve extreme calorie restriction or cutting out entire food groups, which may lead to short-term weight loss but are unsustainable and unhealthy in the long run.

Most of the weight lost on these fad diets is water weight or muscle mass, rather than fat. Once you return to normal eating habits, the weight is often regained, sometimes with additional pounds. Sustainable weight loss is about adopting healthy, balanced eating habits that you can maintain over time—not depriving yourself of essential nutrients.

How to Make Healthier Choices Without Sacrifice

Making healthier choices doesn't have to mean sacrificing the foods and activities you love. In fact, adopting healthier habits can be about balance, moderation, and small changes that add up over time. Instead of viewing healthy living as a restrictive or joyless pursuit, it's important to approach it as a way to enhance your life while still enjoying the things you care about. Here's how you can make healthier choices without feeling like you're giving anything up.

1. Start with Small Changes

A common mistake when trying to live healthier is attempting drastic changes all at once. This often leads to burnout or feelings of deprivation. Instead, focus on small, sustainable changes that you can incorporate gradually. For example, rather than cutting out all sugary snacks immediately, try swapping out one soda for sparkling water or replacing a sugary treat with a piece of fruit a few times a week. These small changes are easier to maintain and won't feel like a big sacrifice.

You can also make slight adjustments to your favorite meals instead of eliminating them. Love pizza? Try adding more vegetables as toppings or opting for a whole-grain crust. Enjoy pasta? Use whole-wheat pasta or a veggie-based alternative like zucchini noodles to increase fiber and reduce processed carbs.

2. Focus on Addition, Not Subtraction

A great way to improve your health without feeling deprived is by focusing on adding nutritious foods to your diet rather than simply cutting things out. For instance, add more fruits and vegetables to your meals, aiming to fill half of your plate with them. When you focus on adding nutrient-dense foods like lean proteins, whole grains, and healthy fats, you naturally crowd out less nutritious options without feeling restricted.

This approach doesn't just apply to food. You can enhance your health by adding more physical activity to your daily routine in ways that are enjoyable and easy to fit in. For example, you don't have to give up screen time to get moving—try exercising while watching TV, or add a short walk during your lunch break. Small additions like these can have a big impact over time.

3. Practice Mindful Eating

Mindful eating is another powerful strategy for making healthier choices without feeling deprived. This involves paying closer attention to what you're eating, how much, and why. Instead of eating while distracted—like in front of the TV—take the time to savor your food. Eat slowly, chew thoroughly, and enjoy the flavors and textures. This can help you feel more satisfied with smaller portions and reduce mindless overeating.

Mindful eating also helps you become more aware of your body's hunger and fullness cues, making it easier to stop eating when you're satisfied rather than stuffed. Over time, this practice can lead to healthier portion control without feeling like you're limiting yourself.

4. Choose Healthier Versions of Your Favorite Foods

Another way to stay healthy without feeling like you're sacrificing anything is by opting for healthier versions of the foods you already love. Craving something sweet? Opt for dark chocolate instead of milk chocolate, which is higher in antioxidants and lower in sugar. If you love fried foods, try air-frying or baking instead of deep-frying to reduce unhealthy fats without sacrificing flavor.

Additionally, you can experiment with healthier cooking methods, such as grilling, steaming, or roasting, instead of frying or using heavy sauces. These simple swaps help you retain the flavors and textures you enjoy while improving the nutritional value of your meals.

5. Allow for Flexibility and Enjoy Treats in Moderation

Healthy living doesn't mean you have to give up your favorite indulgences entirely. In fact, allowing yourself the occasional treat can prevent feelings of deprivation and make it easier to stick to healthier habits in the long term. The key is moderation—enjoying treats mindfully and without guilt.

Instead of aiming for perfection, focus on balance. It's okay to have a slice of cake at a celebration or to enjoy a night out at a restaurant. The important thing is to make healthier choices most of the time and allow for flexibility when needed. This approach makes healthy living feel more sustainable and less restrictive.

Conclusion

Understanding the basics of nutrition—calories, macronutrients, and micronutrients—can empower you to make smarter food choices that fuel your body effectively. Calories provide essential energy, while macronutrients like proteins, carbohydrates, and fats are the building blocks for growth, energy, and maintenance. Micronutrients, although needed in smaller quantities, play a vital role in keeping your body functioning optimally. A balanced diet rich in these nutrients supports overall health, fitness, and weight management goals. However, many myths and misconceptions about dieting and weight loss can derail progress. There are no shortcuts for lasting weight loss—carbohydrates, fats, and even moderate exercise all have a role in a healthy lifestyle. Success lies in understanding your body's needs and maintaining a sustainable, long-term approach.

Making healthier choices doesn't have to feel like a struggle or involve giving up the things you love. Start with small, manageable changes, focus on adding nutritious foods rather than subtracting them, practice mindful eating, and choose healthier versions of your favorite foods. By embracing balance and flexibility, you can create a lifestyle that supports your well-being without sacrificing enjoyment. Remember, health is about progress, not perfection—enjoy the journey while making choices that align with your goals for lasting health.

Chapter 2

Fueling Your Body Right

The Role of Protein, Fats, and Carbs in Weight Loss

When it comes to weight loss, understanding the role of protein, fats, and carbohydrates is crucial for creating a balanced, effective diet plan. These macronutrients play different but essential roles in your body, providing energy, supporting metabolism, and maintaining muscle mass. By consuming the right types of each in the right proportions, you can fuel your weight loss efforts without sacrificing nutrition or overall health.

Protein: The Building Block of Weight Loss

Protein is one of the most important macronutrients for weight loss due to its multiple roles in metabolism, muscle maintenance, and appetite control. Consuming enough protein helps preserve lean muscle mass while losing fat, which is key for long-term weight management. Muscle tissue burns more calories at rest than fat, so maintaining muscle through adequate protein intake keeps your metabolism active even when you're in a calorie deficit.

Additionally, protein has a high thermic effect of food (TEF), meaning your body uses more energy to digest it compared to fats or carbohydrates. This can slightly boost your metabolism and increase the number of calories you burn throughout the day.

Protein is also highly satiating, which helps control appetite and reduce cravings. By incorporating lean sources of protein like chicken, fish, eggs, tofu, and legumes into your diet, you're more likely to feel full and satisfied, reducing the urge to overeat or snack on unhealthy foods.

Fats: Essential for Health and Weight Loss

Fats often get a bad reputation when it comes to weight loss, but they are essential for your body to function properly. Healthy fats, such as those found in avocados, nuts, seeds, olive oil, and fatty fish, are crucial for hormone regulation, including hormones that control hunger and metabolism. Fats also help your body absorb fat-soluble vitamins (A, D, E, and K) and provide long-lasting energy.

Fats are more calorie-dense than protein and carbohydrates, with 9 calories per gram compared to 4 calories per gram for the other two macronutrients. However, because fats are slower to digest, they help keep you full and satisfied for longer periods. This makes it easier to stick to a reduced-calorie diet without feeling deprived.

The key is to focus on healthy, unsaturated fats while limiting saturated and trans fats, which can contribute to weight gain and increase the risk of heart disease. Incorporating sources like olive oil, nuts, and fatty fish into your diet can provide the health benefits of fat without contributing to excessive calorie intake.

Carbohydrates: Fuel for Energy and Performance

Carbohydrates are your body's primary source of energy, especially during physical activity. While some diets advocate for cutting carbs, it's important to remember that not all carbs are created equal. Complex carbohydrates, such as whole grains, vegetables, and legumes, are rich in fiber, vitamins, and minerals. These carbs digest slowly, providing steady energy and helping to keep you full.

Fiber, a type of carbohydrate, plays a significant role in weight loss by promoting healthy digestion and regulating blood sugar levels. High-fiber foods like oats, beans, and leafy greens keep you fuller longer, helping to curb hunger and prevent overeating.

On the other hand, simple carbohydrates, such as refined sugars and white bread, can cause rapid spikes in blood sugar, followed by crashes that lead to hunger and cravings. To support weight loss, focus on consuming complex carbs and fiber-rich foods, while minimizing refined sugars and processed carbohydrates.

Portion Control: Eating the Right Amount Without Counting Every Calorie

Portion control is a key factor in maintaining a healthy diet and achieving weight loss goals without the stress of counting every single calorie. Instead of meticulously tracking calorie intake, focusing on portion sizes allows you to eat the right amount of food to fuel your body while preventing overeating. Learning how to manage portion sizes can help create a balanced, sustainable approach to nutrition that promotes long-term health.

Why Portion Control Matters

Portion sizes have increased significantly in recent years, especially in restaurant servings and packaged foods. This has contributed to overeating and excess calorie consumption, which can lead to weight gain. Many people don't realize they're eating more than they need because the portions we're accustomed to seeing are often much larger than what our bodies require.

By practicing portion control, you can avoid consuming extra calories that may not be necessary for your energy needs. It's about eating mindfully—recognizing when you're satisfied rather than eating until you're overly full. This not only helps with weight management but also encourages healthier eating habits overall.

Simple Tips for Portion Control

1. **Use Smaller Plates and Bowls** One of the simplest ways to control portions is by using smaller plates and bowls. Studies have shown that people tend to eat less when they serve themselves on smaller dishes. The psychology behind this is simple: smaller plates make portions look larger, tricking your brain into feeling satisfied with less food.

2. **Pay Attention to Serving Sizes** Familiarize yourself with recommended serving sizes for common foods. For example, a serving of meat should be roughly the size of a deck of cards, while a serving of pasta is about the size of a tennis ball. Understanding these visual cues can help you keep portions in check without needing to measure or weigh everything.

3. **Fill Half Your Plate with Vegetables** Vegetables are low in calories and high in nutrients, making them a great choice for filling up your plate. By making half of your meal vegetables, you automatically reduce the calorie density of your meal while still feeling full. Leafy greens, broccoli, carrots, and bell peppers are excellent options to bulk up your meal without adding many calories.

4. **Be Mindful of Liquid Calories** Beverages can be a hidden source of extra calories, especially sugary drinks like soda, juice, and alcohol. Drinking water, unsweetened tea, or black coffee instead can help you avoid unnecessary calorie intake. If you're going to enjoy a higher-calorie beverage, be mindful of portion sizes and consider drinking smaller amounts.

5. **Avoid Eating Straight from the Package** It's easy to lose track of how much you're eating when you snack directly from a bag or box. Instead, portion out a serving onto a plate or bowl so you can see exactly how much you're eating. This helps prevent mindless snacking, which can quickly add up in calories.

6. **Slow Down and Listen to Your Body** Eating more slowly allows your brain to catch up with your stomach and recognize when you're full. It takes about 20 minutes for your brain to receive signals of fullness, so slowing down your eating can prevent overeating. Chew thoroughly, savor each bite, and give yourself time to notice when you're satisfied.

Benefits of Portion Control Without Calorie Counting

One of the main advantages of portion control is that it takes the stress out of constantly counting calories. Rather than focusing on numbers, portion control emphasizes mindful eating and making healthier choices. This approach encourages a healthier relationship with food, where you can enjoy meals without feeling restricted or overwhelmed by calorie counts.

Additionally, portion control can help with weight loss and weight maintenance. By consistently eating the right amount of food for your body's needs, you can avoid overeating and create a natural calorie deficit that supports weight loss.

Meal Timing and Metabolism: What Science Says

Meal timing has become a topic of interest in nutrition science, particularly for its effects on metabolism, weight management, and overall health. While the quality and quantity of food are crucial for health, when you eat can also play a significant role in how efficiently your body processes and uses energy. Scientific research suggests that meal timing may influence metabolic rate, hormone release, and how the body stores or burns fat, making it a useful factor to consider for those looking to optimize their metabolism and support a balanced lifestyle.

The Impact of Circadian Rhythms on Metabolism

Our bodies operate on a 24-hour internal clock known as the circadian rhythm, which regulates various physiological functions, including metabolism. Research shows that metabolic processes, such as digestion, insulin sensitivity, and fat oxidation, can fluctuate based on the time of day. In general, our bodies are more efficient at processing food earlier in the day when metabolism is naturally higher. This is why some experts recommend eating larger meals during the morning and afternoon while having lighter meals in the evening.

The Science Behind Breakfast and Metabolism

Breakfast is often emphasized as an important meal to "kickstart" the metabolism, and there's evidence to support this. Eating a nutrient-rich breakfast can stimulate thermogenesis, a process where the body produces heat by burning calories. Studies suggest that breakfast eaters may have better blood sugar control, lower appetite throughout the day, and reduced cravings for unhealthy snacks. Consuming protein, fiber, and healthy fats in the morning can help curb hunger and reduce the likelihood of overeating later in the day.

However, recent research also shows that breakfast might not be essential for everyone, and its impact on metabolism can vary based on individual lifestyle and genetics. Intermittent fasting, for example, is an eating pattern that often involves skipping breakfast, and some studies indicate that it can benefit metabolism and weight management for certain people. Ultimately, the importance of breakfast may come down to personal preference and lifestyle needs.

Eating Frequency and Metabolism

Some people believe that eating small, frequent meals throughout the day helps "boost" metabolism, but research on this is mixed. While eating every few hours can help some individuals avoid hunger and maintain steady energy levels, it doesn't necessarily increase metabolic rate. The thermic effect of food (TEF)—the energy used to digest, absorb, and metabolize food—remains relatively constant regardless of how often you eat. Therefore, meal frequency may be less important for metabolism than the overall balance and quality of your daily food intake.

The Role of Late-Night Eating

Late-night eating is often associated with weight gain and metabolic disruption. Research suggests that eating late at night can interfere with your body's circadian rhythm, resulting in slower digestion, reduced insulin sensitivity, and increased fat storage. When calories are consumed closer to bedtime, they are more likely to be stored as fat rather than burned as energy. For this reason, many nutritionists recommend finishing your last meal several hours before going to sleep to allow for optimal digestion and metabolic function.

Practical Takeaways for Meal Timing and Metabolism

1. **Front-Load Your Calories:** Consuming more of your daily calories earlier in the day can support your natural

metabolic rhythm, helping you feel energized and reducing the likelihood of nighttime hunger.

2. **Personalize Meal Timing:** Meal timing may be best tailored to your lifestyle, work schedule, and personal preferences. For instance, intermittent fasting can be effective for those who find it fits their daily routine without creating excessive hunger.

3. **Avoid Late-Night Meals:** Limiting late-night eating can support better digestion, metabolism, and sleep quality, which in turn may help with weight management.

Conclusion

For successful weight loss, it's essential to balance your intake of protein, fats, and carbohydrates rather than eliminating any one group. Protein helps maintain muscle mass and control appetite, fats provide necessary nutrients and keep you satisfied, and carbohydrates fuel your body for daily activities and exercise. A balanced diet emphasizing whole, nutrient-dense foods not only supports weight loss but also promotes overall health and well-being. Portion control is another effective strategy, helping you enjoy balanced, satisfying meals without needing to count every calorie. By focusing on serving sizes, using smaller plates, and paying attention to hunger cues, you can manage weight in a healthy way and cultivate a positive relationship with food.

Meal timing also plays a significant role in metabolic health. Research suggests that aligning your eating habits with your natural circadian rhythm can benefit metabolism and overall energy levels. Eating larger meals earlier in the day, reducing excessive snacking, and finishing your last meal a few hours before bed are small but impactful changes that can support weight management and metabolic function. By personalizing meal timing and focusing on nutrient-dense foods, you create a diet that sustains energy, supports weight loss goals, and enhances your well-being.

While there's no one-size-fits-all answer to meal timing and metabolism, science suggests that aligning your eating habits with your natural circadian rhythm and focusing on nutrient-dense foods can be beneficial. Eating larger meals earlier in the day, avoiding excessive snacking, and finishing your last meal a few hours before bed are small changes that can have a positive impact on metabolic health. By experimenting with meal timing and listening to your body's needs, you can develop an eating schedule that supports both your metabolism and overall well-being.

Chapter 3

Superfoods and Meal Planning

<u>Superfoods for Weight Loss: What Works and Why</u>

Superfoods have gained popularity for their dense nutritional profiles and potential health benefits, particularly for weight loss. Unlike fad diets or restrictive eating plans, superfoods offer vitamins, minerals, fiber, and antioxidants that support metabolism, energy levels, and overall health. Including these nutrient-dense foods in a balanced diet can enhance your weight loss efforts by keeping you full, satisfied, and energized.

Leafy Greens: Low-Calorie, High-Fiber Nutritional Powerhouses

Leafy greens like spinach, kale, and Swiss chard are excellent for weight loss. These greens are very low in calories but high in fiber, which helps control hunger by slowing digestion and promoting a feeling of fullness. Fiber also supports digestion and gut health, which is important for effective nutrient absorption and metabolism. Leafy greens are also rich in antioxidants, vitamins A and C, and minerals like magnesium and calcium, which support energy levels and immune function.

Berries: Antioxidant-Rich and Naturally Sweet

Berries, such as strawberries, blueberries, and raspberries, are packed with antioxidants that combat oxidative stress, which can improve cellular health and metabolism. They are naturally sweet and low in calories, making them a great alternative to sugary snacks. Their high fiber content aids in stabilizing blood sugar levels, which is key for preventing insulin spikes that can lead to fat storage. Plus, the vitamins and minerals in berries support overall health, helping you stay energized and motivated on your weight loss journey.

Lean Protein Sources: Promoting Satiety and Muscle Maintenance

Lean protein sources like chicken, fish, tofu, and legumes are essential for weight loss. Protein has a high thermic effect, meaning the body uses more energy to digest it compared to fats and carbs, which can boost calorie burn. Protein also supports muscle maintenance, which is important because muscle tissue burns more calories at rest than fat tissue. Including protein in your meals can help control appetite by keeping you full for longer, reducing the likelihood of overeating or snacking on less nutritious options.

Avocado: Healthy Fats for Satiety and Nutrient Absorption

Though high in calories, avocados are rich in monounsaturated fats, which can increase satiety and help control hunger. Healthy fats slow down digestion and provide steady energy, keeping blood sugar levels stable. Additionally, avocados contain fiber, vitamins E and K, potassium, and magnesium, which benefit heart health, reduce inflammation, and improve nutrient absorption. Including a moderate amount of avocado in your meals can make a big difference in satisfaction and prevent cravings.

Green Tea: Boosting Metabolism and Fat Oxidation

Green tea is known for its metabolism-boosting properties, thanks to its caffeine and catechins, which can increase calorie burn and fat oxidation. Studies suggest that drinking green tea regularly may aid in weight loss by promoting thermogenesis—the process of burning calories to produce heat. Green tea is also low in calories, making it a great alternative to sugary beverages. A cup or two per day can support your weight loss goals without adding extra calories.

Chia Seeds: High in Fiber and Omega-3 Fatty Acids

Chia seeds are tiny but powerful superfoods for weight loss. High in fiber, they absorb liquid and expand in the stomach, which can enhance feelings of fullness. This high fiber content also helps regulate blood sugar levels, preventing energy crashes and cravings. Additionally, chia seeds are a good source of omega-3 fatty acids, which reduce inflammation and support heart health. Adding chia seeds to smoothies, yogurt, or oatmeal is a simple way to increase satiety and add nutrients to your diet.

The Importance of Fiber and Hydration

Fiber and hydration are two essential yet often overlooked components of a successful weight loss plan. While diets tend to focus on macronutrients like protein, fats, and carbohydrates, fiber and water play crucial roles in supporting digestion, managing appetite, and optimizing metabolism. Incorporating adequate fiber and hydration into your routine can help you stay full, prevent overeating, and ultimately make it easier to reach your weight loss goals.

The Role of Fiber in Weight Loss

Fiber is a type of carbohydrate that the body can't digest, allowing it to pass through the digestive system largely intact. There are two types of fiber—soluble and insoluble—each with distinct benefits. Soluble fiber dissolves in water to form a gel-like substance, which slows digestion and helps stabilize blood sugar levels. This type of fiber is found in foods like oats, apples, and legumes. Insoluble fiber, found in whole grains, vegetables, and seeds, adds bulk to stool, promoting regular bowel movements and supporting gut health.

One of the primary ways fiber aids in weight loss is by enhancing feelings of fullness, or satiety. Foods high in fiber tend to take longer to chew and digest, which helps reduce the likelihood of overeating by giving your body more time to signal that it's full. Additionally, fiber-rich foods usually have a lower calorie density, meaning they provide fewer calories per gram compared to high-fat or high-sugar foods. As a result, you can eat a larger volume of food without consuming excess calories, making it easier to stick to a calorie-controlled diet.

Fiber also helps regulate blood sugar by slowing the absorption of glucose into the bloodstream. This prevents the rapid spikes and crashes in blood sugar that can trigger hunger and cravings, particularly for sugary foods. By stabilizing blood sugar levels, fiber can support energy levels and reduce the urge to snack on unhealthy options, further supporting weight loss efforts.

The Importance of Hydration for Weight Loss

Water is fundamental for nearly every bodily function, including digestion, circulation, temperature regulation, and waste elimination. When it comes to weight loss, staying well-hydrated can support these processes and make it easier to manage your appetite and energy levels. Dehydration can often mimic feelings of hunger, leading people to eat when they're actually thirsty. By drinking water regularly throughout the day, you can prevent confusion between hunger and thirst and avoid unnecessary snacking.

Drinking water before meals can also help with portion control. Studies show that consuming a glass of water before eating can increase feelings of fullness, helping you eat fewer calories at the meal. Water-rich foods like fruits and vegetables contribute to hydration as well and are often low in calories while high in fiber, making them excellent additions to a weight loss-friendly diet.

Hydration is also essential for proper metabolism and fat oxidation. Water helps transport nutrients to cells and plays a role in breaking down stored fat for energy. Without enough water, these metabolic processes slow down, making it harder to burn calories efficiently. Additionally, water aids in removing waste products from the body through urine and sweat, which is important for maintaining optimal energy levels and preventing bloating.

How Fiber and Hydration Work Together

Fiber and water work in tandem to promote digestive health. For instance, fiber needs water to function effectively in the digestive tract. Soluble fiber absorbs water to form the gel that slows digestion, while insoluble fiber requires water to soften stool and prevent constipation. By ensuring you consume adequate water along with fiber-rich foods, you can maximize the digestive benefits of both and support smoother, more regular bowel movements.

Meal Prepping for Success: Tips and Recipes

Meal prepping is a powerful strategy for achieving your health and weight loss goals, helping you save time, reduce stress, and maintain control over your diet. By planning and preparing meals ahead of time, you can make healthy eating more convenient and avoid the temptation of last-minute, less nutritious options. With a few smart tips and simple recipes, meal prepping can become an enjoyable and sustainable habit that supports long-term success.

Why Meal Prepping Works

When life gets busy, healthy eating can often take a backseat. Meal prepping allows you to stay on track by having nutritious, balanced meals readily available. Preparing meals in advance not only reduces the need for takeout or fast food but also helps you manage portions, control calorie intake, and limit added sugars or unhealthy fats. It's also cost-effective, as buying ingredients in bulk and cooking at home is often less expensive than eating out. Additionally, meal prepping reduces food waste, as you plan only for what you'll actually use.

Tips for Effective Meal Prepping

1. **Plan Your Meals and Snacks**: Start by deciding how many meals you need for the week. Consider breakfast, lunch, dinner, and any snacks. Choose recipes that incorporate a balance of protein, healthy fats, and complex carbohydrates to keep you full and energized.
2. **Choose Simple, Versatile Recipes**: Opt for recipes that are easy to cook in large batches and can be stored well in the fridge or freezer. Dishes like stir-fries, salads, soups,

and grain bowls are versatile, making it easy to mix and match flavors throughout the week.

3. **Invest in Quality Containers**: Using reusable containers that are microwave- and freezer-safe can make meal prep easier and more organized. Divided containers are also helpful for portion control and keeping ingredients fresh.

4. **Set Aside a Prep Day**: Choose a specific day each week, like Sunday, to prepare your meals. Dedicate a few hours to chopping, cooking, and assembling dishes for the week. By having a consistent prep day, meal prepping becomes part of your routine.

5. **Organize Your Ingredients**: Start by prepping ingredients that require longer cooking times, like grains or proteins, while you chop vegetables or prepare dressings. This saves time and ensures that everything is ready at the same time.

6. **Store Meals Properly**: Proper storage is key to keeping meals fresh. Most prepared meals last around 3-5 days in the fridge. For longer storage, freeze portions in airtight containers and defrost as needed.

Easy Meal Prep Recipes

1. **Overnight Oats**: Combine ½ cup rolled oats, 1 cup milk or a dairy-free alternative, and toppings like berries, nuts, or chia seeds in a jar. Refrigerate overnight for a quick, nutritious breakfast.

2. **Chicken and Veggie Stir-Fry**: Sauté chicken breast slices with mixed veggies like bell peppers, broccoli, and snap peas in olive oil. Season with garlic, ginger, and low-sodium soy sauce. Serve with brown rice or quinoa, and store portions in individual containers.

3. **Quinoa Salad Bowls**: Combine cooked quinoa with chopped cucumbers, cherry tomatoes, chickpeas, and spinach. Add a simple dressing of olive oil, lemon juice, and herbs for a healthy, filling meal.

4. **Vegetable Soup**: Cook a batch of vegetable soup using carrots, celery, zucchini, tomatoes, and your favorite broth. Add lentils or beans for protein. This soup stores well in the fridge and can be easily reheated.
5. **Energy Bites**: For a quick snack, mix rolled oats, peanut butter, honey, and dark chocolate chips. Form into small balls and refrigerate. These energy bites are perfect for when you need a quick boost.

Conclusion

Superfoods like leafy greens, berries, lean proteins, avocados, green tea, and chia seeds offer essential nutrients that can support weight loss by controlling hunger, boosting metabolism, and providing sustained energy. When incorporated into a balanced diet, these nutrient-dense foods make it easier to maintain healthy eating habits without extreme restrictions. By focusing on foods that nourish and satisfy, you're more likely to achieve and sustain your weight loss goals.

Additionally, adequate fiber and hydration play crucial roles in supporting a healthy metabolism and managing appetite. Fiber-rich foods help regulate blood sugar, promote satiety, and aid digestion, while staying hydrated helps prevent overeating, keeps energy levels stable, and supports metabolic function. Together, fiber and water create a sustainable eating approach that contributes to long-term weight management and overall health.

Meal prepping can further simplify healthy eating by providing ready-made, nutritious options, even during busy times. With a bit of planning, meal prep ensures balanced meals are always within reach, helping you stay on track with your wellness goals. By organizing meals ahead of time, you gain control over portions and ingredients, making healthy living a more convenient and enjoyable routine.

Chapter 4

Managing Cravings and Emotional Eating

Understanding Cravings: What Your Body is Really Asking For

Cravings can feel like they appear out of nowhere, urging us to reach for specific foods—often high-calorie, sugary, or salty options. But beneath these impulses, our bodies may actually be signaling deeper needs. Understanding cravings allows you to respond with mindfulness and care, often making choices that better satisfy your body and prevent overeating or emotional eating. Here's an in-depth look at what your body may be communicating through cravings and how to interpret these signals.

Cravings and Nutritional Deficiencies

Many cravings stem from unmet nutritional needs, as the body sometimes signals a specific food when it needs certain vitamins or minerals. For instance:

- **Chocolate Cravings**: Chocolate cravings may indicate a magnesium deficiency, as chocolate, particularly dark chocolate, is high in magnesium. Magnesium supports muscle function, stress reduction, and even sleep quality. To meet this need without relying on chocolate, you might add magnesium-rich foods like nuts, seeds, leafy greens, and bananas to your diet.
- **Salty Cravings**: A craving for salty foods could signal a need for sodium or other electrolytes, especially after sweating a lot through exercise or hot weather. Sodium is essential for fluid balance and nerve function, but rather than reaching for processed salty snacks, consider a more

balanced source of sodium, like pickled vegetables or nuts, or simply stay well-hydrated with water and electrolyte sources.

- **Carbohydrate Cravings**: The body might signal a need for carbohydrates when energy levels are low, as carbs are its primary fuel source. This craving is often intensified when you're under-eating or over-exercising. Instead of reaching for refined carbs, try complex carbohydrates like whole grains, vegetables, and fruits, which offer sustained energy and fiber.

Recognizing these cravings as potential signals of nutrient needs empowers you to choose healthier, nutrient-dense alternatives that satisfy your body.

Emotional Cravings: Finding Comfort and Balance

Cravings are also heavily influenced by emotional states, as many people turn to food for comfort or stress relief. Stress, sadness, boredom, loneliness, or even excitement can all drive cravings, particularly for foods that are high in sugar and fat. These foods trigger the release of dopamine, a "feel-good" neurotransmitter, providing a temporary mood boost. However, this response is short-lived, often leading to more cravings or regret afterward.

By identifying emotional eating triggers, you can begin to respond in healthier ways. For instance:

- **If you crave sugary foods during stress**: This could be a sign that you're seeking comfort or energy during tough times. Rather than sugary snacks, consider stress-relief alternatives like a quick walk, a few deep breaths, or a relaxing hobby. These non-food actions can often relieve stress without the crash that follows a sugar high.
- **If you eat out of boredom or loneliness**: Filling the need for connection or stimulation in other ways—calling a friend, engaging in a hobby, or even journaling—can

help satisfy the craving for food with something that truly nourishes your emotional needs.

When you identify the emotional triggers behind cravings, you'll be better equipped to replace the habit of emotional eating with healthier, more satisfying activities.

Habitual and Environmental Cravings

Our environment, routines, and habits also play a huge role in the cravings we experience. Repeated behaviors, like always having a snack during a TV show or associating certain activities with food, can become conditioned responses, prompting cravings regardless of hunger. Environmental cues, like seeing others eat or passing by a favorite bakery, can also trigger cravings.

To manage these habitual cravings:

- **Change Your Routine**: If you're used to snacking while watching TV, try substituting that snack with herbal tea or another relaxing activity. Over time, you'll break the association between snacking and the activity.
- **Manage Your Environment**: Keep healthy snacks accessible and avoid storing tempting treats in visible or easy-to-reach places. This small change can help you reach for nutrient-dense foods over impulse-driven options.

By acknowledging these habitual cravings and modifying routines, you'll find it easier to make choices aligned with your health goals rather than automatic habits.

Listening to Your Body's True Needs

Understanding and responding to cravings requires a mix of mindfulness and patience. When a craving strikes, pause and ask yourself a few questions:

1. **Am I hungry, or am I looking to fill another need?** If you're genuinely hungry, choose a nutritious option. If not, consider what you're actually feeling and how you can address that need directly.
2. **What am I craving, and why?** Try to determine whether the craving might be related to a nutrient your body is asking for or if it's connected to an emotional state.
3. **How can I satisfy this craving in a healthier way?** If you crave something sweet, consider fruit or dark chocolate. If you crave something crunchy and salty, try nuts or seeds.

Learning to distinguish between physical and emotional cravings takes practice, but it's a skill that can help you make healthier, more satisfying food choices over time. By understanding your cravings, you'll not only improve your diet but also build a healthier relationship with food, where eating becomes more about nourishment than simply satisfying an impulse.

Emotional Eating: Recognizing and Overcoming Triggers

Emotional eating is a common struggle, where food becomes a response to emotions rather than hunger. Often, people reach for snacks or comfort foods not because their bodies need fuel, but because they're feeling stressed, lonely, bored, anxious, or even happy. Recognizing the triggers behind emotional eating can be the first step toward developing healthier habits and finding ways to meet emotional needs without relying on food. Here's a detailed look at why emotional eating happens, how to recognize your unique triggers, and practical steps to overcome them.

Understanding Emotional Eating and Its Triggers

Emotional eating is tied to the brain's reward system, which releases dopamine—a "feel-good" neurotransmitter—when we eat pleasurable foods, especially those high in sugar and fat. This response creates a temporary sense of relief or comfort, making it easy to associate eating with emotional regulation. Over time, emotional eating can become a habit, with certain situations, feelings, or times of day triggering the urge to eat.

Common triggers for emotional eating include:

1. **Stress:** Stress releases cortisol, a hormone that increases appetite and cravings for high-calorie foods. This response is tied to the body's ancient survival mechanisms, as it anticipates the need for extra energy to face "threats"—even if they're modern stressors like work or relationships.
2. **Boredom:** When there's little mental stimulation, reaching for food can provide a temporary distraction or activity. Boredom eating often fills the gap where engaging activities or connections might be more satisfying.
3. **Sadness and Loneliness:** Food, especially comforting or nostalgic choices, can offer a sense of connection or fill

emotional voids. When we're feeling down or disconnected, eating something pleasurable can feel like self-care, even if it only provides a temporary lift.

4. **Celebration and Social Pressure**: Emotions related to happiness or celebration can also lead to eating even when you're not hungry. Social gatherings often involve food, and cultural norms or peer pressure can create an expectation to eat, whether you need it or not.

Recognizing Your Emotional Eating Triggers

To address emotional eating, it's essential to first identify what situations or emotions tend to make you reach for food. This awareness can help break the automatic response between feeling an emotion and turning to eating.

A few practical steps to recognize your triggers include:

- **Track Your Eating Patterns**: Keep a journal to log what you eat, when, and why. Take note of what you're feeling right before eating, especially when you're not truly hungry. Over time, you may notice patterns revealing specific emotions or times of day when you're more likely to eat emotionally.

- **Pause and Check In with Yourself**: When you feel the urge to eat, pause and ask yourself if you're truly hungry. Hunger often has physical signs, like a growling stomach or a sense of emptiness, while emotional hunger tends to be more urgent and specific, like a craving for a particular food.

- **Rate Your Hunger and Emotions**: On a scale from 1 to 10, rate both your physical hunger and emotional state. If your hunger is low but your emotional intensity is high, this might be a clue that you're eating to cope with feelings rather than to satisfy hunger.

Overcoming Emotional Eating Triggers

Once you're aware of your emotional triggers, the next step is to develop healthier ways to respond. Here are some effective strategies:

1. **Find Non-Food Coping Mechanisms**: Discover activities that provide comfort, distraction, or joy without involving food. Exercise, for example, can be a powerful mood booster. Taking a walk, practicing yoga, journaling, listening to music, or calling a friend can also be satisfying alternatives. When you're aware of what emotions trigger your eating, you can match them with healthier ways to respond.

2. **Practice Mindful Eating**: Mindful eating involves paying full attention to the experience of eating—savoring each bite, noticing flavors, and being present with your food. Practicing mindful eating can help reduce emotional eating, as it encourages you to enjoy food for nourishment rather than as a way to avoid feelings. When you slow down, you're more likely to realize when you're full and to enjoy food more without overeating.

3. **Work Through Emotional Challenges**: If certain emotions consistently lead to emotional eating, consider addressing them through other outlets, like journaling, talking to a friend, or even speaking with a therapist. Emotional eating often masks underlying challenges, and working through them can help you better manage your relationship with food.

4. **Set Boundaries for Food Availability**: Environmental cues can fuel emotional eating, so consider creating boundaries to make impulsive eating less likely. For example, keeping tempting foods out of sight, portioning out snacks instead of eating from the package, or designating certain areas for eating can reduce mindless snacking.

5. **Give Yourself Permission to Feel**: Often, people reach for food to avoid or numb emotions, but letting yourself fully experience these emotions can be transformative. Remind yourself that it's okay to feel stressed, sad, or anxious. Emotions are part of being human, and learning to sit with them can help reduce the impulse to cope through food.

Building a Support System

Emotional eating can feel isolating, but many people experience it. Sharing your journey with others—whether friends, family, or support groups—can provide encouragement and accountability. Knowing you're not alone, and that others also struggle with these habits, can make it easier to develop new responses to emotional triggers.

Practical Strategies to Stay on Track

Staying on track with a balanced diet can be challenging, especially when cravings and emotional eating come into play. Rather than aiming for perfection, a more realistic approach involves practical strategies to manage urges and cultivate a consistent routine. With a few tools and techniques, you can stay aligned with your health goals while learning to navigate cravings and emotions more effectively. Here are some actionable strategies to help you maintain a healthy lifestyle.

1. Plan Ahead

One of the most effective ways to avoid giving in to cravings and emotional eating is by planning your meals and snacks in advance. This doesn't mean you need to rigidly control every bite, but having nutritious options readily available can prevent you from reaching for less healthy choices when hunger or emotions hit. Consider dedicating time once or twice a week to prepare simple, balanced meals. Healthy snacks, like pre-cut veggies, fruits, nuts, or yogurt, can be kept on hand so that you have satisfying options when hunger or cravings strike.

2. Practice Mindful Eating

Mindful eating is a powerful tool for managing cravings and emotional eating. By focusing on your meal without distractions, you can tune in to your body's hunger and fullness signals, allowing you to enjoy food without overeating. Practicing mindful eating involves slowing down, savoring each bite, and paying attention to the taste, texture, and aroma of your food. This technique can help you feel more satisfied with less food and prevent mindless eating that's often fueled by emotions or boredom.

3. Identify Triggers and Build New Habits

Understanding what triggers your cravings or emotional eating habits is crucial. Triggers can be internal (like stress or sadness) or external (such as seeing an ad for a dessert). Once you identify your specific triggers, work on developing healthier habits. For instance, if you find yourself craving sweets when stressed, try deep breathing, a quick walk, or another activity that helps you de-stress without involving food. Building new habits takes time, but each small shift contributes to lasting change.

4. Focus on Balance, Not Restriction

Restrictive diets often lead to stronger cravings, which can result in overeating or bingeing. Instead of cutting out your favorite foods entirely, focus on balance. Allow yourself occasional treats and aim for nutrient-dense foods most of the time. When you allow yourself flexibility, you're less likely to experience strong cravings or feel deprived, making it easier to stay consistent over the long term. You could even try the 80/20 rule: 80% of the time, eat whole, nutritious foods, and allow yourself 20% for the foods you enjoy.

5. Build a Support System

A strong support system can make all the difference when it comes to staying on track. Friends, family members, or online communities with similar goals can provide encouragement, share tips, and help hold you accountable. Sometimes, just talking about your challenges with someone can ease the emotional burden and help you stay focused. If you're comfortable, share your goals with those close to you so they can offer positive support without judgment.

6. Drink Water First

Often, thirst is mistaken for hunger. When you feel a craving coming on, try drinking a glass of water first and wait a few minutes. Staying hydrated not only helps prevent false hunger but also supports digestion, energy levels, and metabolism. Adding a daily hydration habit can also reduce the likelihood of mindless snacking or cravings throughout the day.

7. Set Small, Achievable Goals

Setting small, specific goals can keep you motivated and give you a sense of accomplishment. Instead of aiming for large, overarching goals, start with manageable changes, like eating one extra serving of vegetables daily or choosing fruit over a sugary snack. Each small success helps build confidence, showing you that progress is possible without overwhelming yourself.

8. Reward Yourself Without Food

Sometimes, we turn to food as a reward, which can reinforce emotional eating patterns. Instead, find non-food rewards that bring you joy and relaxation, such as watching a favorite show, reading a book, or indulging in a hobby. Rewarding yourself with activities you love helps shift the focus from food and provides a fulfilling way to celebrate your progress.

Conclusion

Understanding cravings and learning to decode their meaning can be empowering on the path to healthier eating. Rather than viewing cravings as weaknesses, consider them as signals from your body or mind, indicating specific needs—whether for nutrients, comfort, or a shift in routine. By addressing the root causes, you can make mindful choices that truly satisfy you, leading to better health and a more balanced relationship with food. Remember, listening to your body doesn't mean giving in to every craving, but rather responding in ways that support your well-being and long-term goals.

Understanding and overcoming emotional eating is a journey that requires patience and self-compassion. By recognizing your triggers, practicing mindful strategies, and developing healthier responses, you can begin to break the cycle of emotional eating. Instead of turning to food in times of stress or emotional discomfort, you'll gain tools to navigate these emotions more effectively, ultimately leading to a healthier and more balanced relationship with eating.

Staying on track with a healthy eating plan doesn't mean eliminating cravings or emotions but managing them in ways that support your goals. By planning ahead, practicing mindfulness, identifying triggers, and focusing on balanced choices, you can develop a sustainable approach to eating. Incorporating hydration, setting small goals, and rewarding yourself without food also help you build lasting habits that support well-being. These strategies empower you to navigate challenges effectively, making it easier to stay on track in a realistic, enjoyable way.

Chapter 5

Smart Snacking and Eating Out

<u>Healthy Snacks for Sustained Energy</u>

Incorporating healthy snacks into your diet is an effective way to maintain steady energy levels throughout the day and prevent overeating at main meals. Healthy snacks can provide the nutrients you need for sustained energy without leading to energy crashes or unplanned splurges. Here are some key principles for choosing snacks that fuel your body effectively and examples of nutrient-packed options to keep you energized and satisfied.

1. Choose Nutrient-Dense Options

When you're looking to maintain energy, focus on nutrient-dense snacks that combine protein, healthy fats, and complex carbohydrates. This balance provides a steady release of glucose into your bloodstream, which helps keep you feeling alert and focused without the highs and lows of sugar-filled snacks. Protein and healthy fats also play a role in slowing digestion, which prolongs the energy you get from food.

Examples:

- Greek yogurt with fresh berries and a sprinkle of chia seeds
- Hummus with sliced bell peppers, cucumbers, or carrots
- Cottage cheese topped with a handful of nuts and sliced fruit
- Hard-boiled eggs paired with avocado slices

2. Prioritize Fiber for Fullness

Fiber-rich snacks help maintain energy by keeping you fuller for longer and stabilizing blood sugar. Fiber also supports digestive health, which is essential for nutrient absorption and overall energy. Opting for whole grains, vegetables, and fruits with their natural fiber content helps you avoid cravings and hunger spikes.

Examples:

- Apple slices with almond butter
- Whole-grain toast with avocado and cherry tomatoes
- Fresh berries with a sprinkle of ground flaxseed or walnuts
- Oatmeal with a small handful of nuts and a few sliced strawberries

3. Opt for Complex Carbohydrates Over Simple Sugars

Simple sugars cause a rapid spike in blood sugar, followed by a crash that leaves you feeling sluggish. Complex carbohydrates, on the other hand, are digested more slowly, providing sustained energy over time. Whole grains, fruits, and starchy vegetables make excellent choices for a balanced, energizing snack.

Examples:

- Sweet potato wedges sprinkled with cinnamon
- Whole-grain crackers with guacamole or cottage cheese
- Brown rice cakes topped with almond butter and banana slices
- A small portion of trail mix with nuts, seeds, and a few dried cranberries (in moderation)

4. Incorporate Hydration Into Your Snacks

Dehydration can often lead to feelings of fatigue, so consider hydrating snacks as part of your energy-boosting routine. Fruits and vegetables with high water content can help keep you hydrated while delivering vitamins, minerals, and natural sugars for quick energy.

Examples:

- Watermelon or cantaloupe cubes
- Cucumber and mint-infused water with a handful of nuts
- Orange slices with a sprinkle of chia seeds
- Celery sticks with cottage cheese or nut butter

5. Plan Ahead for Smart Snacking Choices

When hunger strikes unexpectedly, have pre-prepared snacks on hand can prevent impulsive choices that may lead to energy crashes. Planning your snacks with a balance of protein, healthy fats, and fiber in mind ensures you'll always have energizing options available.

Examples of Pre-Prepared Snack Packs:

- Snack-size containers of Greek yogurt with a serving of mixed berries
- Small baggies of almonds, walnuts, and a sprinkle of dark chocolate chips
- Mini vegetable packs with hummus or guacamole
- Overnight oats topped with berries and chia seeds

How to Make Smart Choices at Restaurants and Social Events

Making healthy choices at restaurants and social events can be a challenge, as it often involves tempting foods, large portions, and limited control over ingredients. However, by planning ahead, being mindful of your selections, and adopting a few key strategies, you can navigate these situations without compromising your wellness goals. Here's how to make smarter choices when dining out or attending social gatherings, so you can enjoy the experience while staying on track.

1. Look at the Menu in Advance

If possible, preview the restaurant's menu online beforehand. Most restaurants offer detailed menus, including ingredients and nutritional information. By planning your order in advance, you're less likely to make impulsive decisions when you arrive. Look for options that are grilled, baked, steamed, or roasted, as these are generally healthier than fried or sautéed choices. Salads, lean proteins, and whole grains are often good starting points.

Pro Tip: Identify substitutions that might make your meal healthier. For example, you could ask for extra vegetables instead of fries, or request a whole-grain bread option if available.

2. Control Portion Sizes

Restaurant portions are often larger than needed, which can lead to overeating. One helpful strategy is to ask for a half-portion, share a meal with a friend, or immediately set aside half of your plate to take home. Some people find it helpful to order an appetizer as their main course, or to pair a starter salad with a side for a balanced, satisfying meal without overindulging.

Pro Tip: You can also ask for a to-go box when your food arrives and place half your meal in it before you start eating. This way, you won't feel pressured to finish everything on the plate.

3. Be Mindful of Hidden Calories in Sauces and Dressings

Sauces, dressings, and condiments can add unexpected calories, sodium, and sugar to your meal. To manage this, request these items on the side so you can control how much you add. A small amount of dressing or sauce can enhance the flavor without compromising your meal's nutritional value. For salads, vinaigrettes or olive oil and vinegar are generally better choices than creamy dressings.

Pro Tip: If you're ordering something with a sauce or dressing already mixed in, ask if it can be made with less, or see if they offer a lighter version. Even a simple request to "go light" on the dressing can make a difference.

4. Choose Healthier Beverages

Drinks can be a major source of hidden calories, especially at social events or dinners. Soft drinks, cocktails, and specialty coffees often come with high sugar content. Opt for water, sparkling water, unsweetened iced tea, or a light drink such as a wine spritzer. If you want to enjoy a cocktail or glass of wine, consider alternating with water to pace yourself.

Pro Tip: Adding a slice of lemon or lime to water can make it more enjoyable and satisfying. Sparkling water with a splash of juice is another low-calorie alternative to sugary drinks.

5. Focus on Protein and Vegetables

When ordering, aim for a balanced plate by prioritizing lean protein sources and vegetables, which are generally nutrient-dense and lower in calories. Grilled chicken, fish, and plant-based proteins such as beans or lentils are great choices. If you're ordering a pasta dish or a wrap, consider adding a side salad or ordering extra veggies to round out your meal and make it more filling.

Pro Tip: Start your meal with a salad or veggie-based soup. This can curb your hunger and make you less likely to overeat the main course.

6. Pace Yourself and Enjoy the Experience

Eating slowly gives your body time to register fullness, which can help prevent overeating. Take time to savor each bite, enjoy the company, and engage in conversation. By focusing on the experience rather than solely on the food, you'll feel more satisfied and avoid the common habit of eating quickly, which often leads to overeating.

Pro Tip: Put your fork down between bites and take a sip of water. This simple practice can help slow your eating pace and make you more mindful of your food.

7. Make Socializing the Priority

At social events, focus on the people and the occasion rather than just the food. Mingling and talking with others can keep you from mindlessly grazing at the snack table or going back for seconds. Shift your attention to conversations, activities, and enjoying the atmosphere, which can help you manage cravings and make more mindful food choices.

Pro Tip: When you arrive at a social event, take a quick survey of the food options, then decide what's worth having. Pick a few items you genuinely want to enjoy and skip the rest.

Navigating Cravings While Sticking to Your Plan

Navigating cravings while sticking to a healthy eating plan can be challenging, but understanding what causes these urges and having strategies in place can make it easier to manage them. Cravings are often tied to both physical and emotional triggers and may signal anything from a nutritional need to stress, fatigue, or even boredom. Here's how you can recognize cravings, respond to them more effectively, and stay on track with your health goals.

1. Recognize Your Triggers

The first step in managing cravings is identifying what triggers them. Triggers can be internal, like stress or lack of sleep, or external, such as certain environments, times of day, or even social situations. For instance, many people crave sweets when they're feeling stressed or reach for salty snacks when they're bored. When you feel a craving come on, pause and assess what might be causing it. By understanding whether you're genuinely hungry or responding to an emotional or situational trigger, you can make a more conscious choice about whether to satisfy it.

Pro Tip: Keep a food and mood journal for a few days, noting the times you have cravings and what was happening around you. This can help you identify patterns and create strategies for the future.

2. Find Healthier Alternatives

If a craving is hard to ignore, consider satisfying it with a healthier alternative. Craving something sweet? Opt for a piece of fruit, like an apple or berries, which will provide natural sugars along with fiber and vitamins. If you're craving something salty, try a handful of nuts or a few olives, which contain healthy fats that can help you feel more satisfied. This approach allows you to honor your craving without derailing your plan.

Pro Tip: Prepare a list of healthier alternatives for common cravings, so when a craving hits, you have an immediate go-to choice that aligns with your health goals.

3. Practice Mindful Eating

Mindful eating can be incredibly effective in managing cravings. This approach encourages you to slow down, pay attention to your hunger signals, and fully savor each bite. Before reaching for a snack or treat, ask yourself if you're truly hungry or just responding to a craving. If you do decide to eat, do so slowly and enjoy the flavors and textures, which often leads to greater satisfaction with a smaller amount of food.

Pro Tip: When you feel a craving, drink a glass of water and wait 5-10 minutes before deciding if you want to eat. Sometimes, dehydration can be mistaken for hunger or cravings.

4. Plan Satisfying Meals and Snacks

Including filling, balanced meals throughout the day can reduce cravings. Focus on meals that combine protein, fiber, and healthy fats, as this combination helps stabilize blood sugar and maintain energy levels, making it less likely for cravings to arise. Additionally, planning for healthy snacks can give you satisfying options when you need a boost, helping you avoid impulse choices.

Pro Tip: Prepare a few high-protein or high-fiber snacks, like Greek yogurt with berries or carrot sticks with hummus, so you always have something filling and nutritious on hand.

5. Allow Yourself Small Indulgences

Trying to completely avoid all treats can make cravings stronger. Allowing yourself a small portion of a favorite food every now and then can help you feel more satisfied and reduce the risk of bingeing. The key is moderation—enjoy a small square of dark chocolate, a few chips, or a single scoop of ice cream if you really want it. This way, you can savor a treat without losing control.

Pro Tip: Schedule your indulgences. Knowing you have a treat planned, like a dessert on the weekend or a fun snack once a week, can make it easier to avoid mindless snacking during the week.

6. Use Distraction Techniques

Sometimes, cravings will pass if you simply redirect your attention. When a craving strikes, find an activity that can occupy your mind and body. A short walk, a puzzle, a phone call with a friend, or even a few minutes of deep breathing exercises can shift your focus away from the craving and onto something more productive. Distraction can be particularly helpful with emotional cravings, as it reduces the association between difficult emotions and food.

Pro Tip: Keep a list of quick, enjoyable activities you can turn to when a craving hits. This helps create a positive routine that isn't food-focused.

Final Thoughts

Making healthy snacking choices allows you to sustain your energy levels, prevent hunger-induced fatigue, and stay focused throughout the day. By selecting nutrient-dense, fiber-rich, and hydrating snacks, you're supporting your body's need for energy and satisfying your hunger in a balanced, sustainable way. The more thoughtful and prepared you are about your snacking choices, the more you'll be able to maintain consistent energy and avoid the pitfalls of quick-fix, sugary options.

Eating at restaurants and social events can still align with your health and wellness goals if you approach these situations with mindful planning and a few smart strategies. By planning ahead, controlling portions, making thoughtful substitutions, and focusing on protein and vegetables, you'll be better equipped to make healthy choices without feeling restricted.

Part 2

Exercise for a Fit and Strong Body

Chapter 6

The Role of Exercise in Weight Loss

<u>Why Exercise Matters for Fat Loss and Overall Health</u>

Exercise is a powerful tool for achieving fat loss and enhancing overall health. While diet plays a central role in weight management, exercise amplifies the fat-burning process, increases metabolism, and offers numerous benefits that support a healthy body and mind. Understanding why exercise matters for fat loss and general well-being can help individuals make exercise a priority in their daily lives and experience transformative results beyond just the scale.

1. Boosting Metabolism and Burning Calories

Exercise helps increase the number of calories the body burns each day. This is crucial for fat loss, as the body must be in a calorie deficit—burning more calories than it consumes—to reduce fat. Activities like cardio, high-intensity interval training (HIIT), and resistance training accelerate calorie expenditure both during and after exercise, a phenomenon known as the "afterburn effect." When you engage in intense activities, your body's metabolism remains elevated for hours afterward, allowing it to burn more calories even at rest.

Muscle tissue also plays a role here, as it requires more energy to maintain than fat tissue. Through strength training exercises, you can increase your lean muscle mass, which further boosts resting metabolism. With a higher resting metabolic rate, your body becomes more efficient at burning calories, leading to gradual, sustainable fat loss.

2. Reducing Body Fat and Preserving Lean Muscle

Effective fat loss focuses on reducing body fat while maintaining or even building lean muscle. Diet alone can lead to weight loss, but without exercise, the body might lose muscle mass along with fat. This not only slows down metabolism but can also make it harder to maintain weight loss in the long run.

Exercise, particularly resistance and strength training, preserves lean muscle during calorie deficits, helping to achieve a "toned" appearance as fat is lost. This muscle maintenance not only enhances body composition but also prevents the drop in metabolic rate that often comes with dieting. As a result, exercise supports a healthier, leaner physique without sacrificing muscle, making fat loss more sustainable.

3. Improving Cardiovascular and Overall Health

Exercise strengthens the heart and improves cardiovascular health, which is vital for overall well-being and longevity. Regular physical activity enhances circulation, reduces blood pressure, and lowers the risk of chronic conditions like heart disease, diabetes, and stroke. Aerobic exercises such as walking, running, swimming, and cycling strengthen the cardiovascular system, while strength training supports heart health by improving blood flow and reducing bad cholesterol levels.

Additionally, regular exercise benefits brain health. Physical activity has been linked to improved mood, memory, and cognitive function, due to its impact on hormones such as serotonin and endorphins. Exercise also reduces stress levels, a key factor in preventing emotional eating, which can contribute to weight gain.

4. Enhancing Energy Levels and Mood

While exercise may seem tiring at first, it actually boosts energy levels in the long term. Physical activity increases blood flow and oxygen levels in the body, leading to higher energy and alertness throughout the day. Exercise also helps regulate hormones, making you feel happier and more balanced. These mood-boosting effects are essential, as they improve mental resilience and motivation, which are key for sticking to a weight loss journey.

5. Developing Consistency for Sustainable Fat Loss

Consistency is vital for sustainable fat loss. Exercise not only helps with immediate calorie burn but also fosters a routine that reinforces healthy habits over time. When combined with a balanced diet, consistent exercise creates a lifestyle that promotes long-term health, making it easier to maintain a healthy weight and prevent future weight regain.

Incorporating exercise that you enjoy is crucial for sustaining this consistency. Whether it's dancing, hiking, yoga, or weightlifting, find activities that you look forward to doing. This makes staying active a natural part of your lifestyle, rather than a chore.

Cardio vs. Strength Training: What's More Effective?

When it comes to weight loss, two types of exercise typically take the spotlight: cardio and strength training. Both approaches play unique roles in supporting fat loss, boosting metabolism, and improving overall health. Understanding the benefits of each and how to incorporate them effectively can maximize your results and support a balanced, sustainable fitness routine.

Benefits of Cardio for Weight Loss

Cardiovascular exercises, or cardio, include activities like running, cycling, swimming, and brisk walking, which elevate the heart rate for extended periods. The primary advantage of cardio is its ability to burn a significant number of calories in a relatively short amount of time. Regular cardio sessions help create a calorie deficit, which is essential for weight loss. In addition, cardio exercises improve cardiovascular health by strengthening the heart and lungs, reducing the risk of diseases such as hypertension, high cholesterol, and certain heart conditions.

High-Intensity Interval Training (HIIT), a form of cardio, has become increasingly popular for its fat-burning potential. HIIT workouts involve short, intense bursts of exercise followed by recovery periods, which can significantly elevate calorie burn in a shorter period compared to steady-state cardio. Plus, HIIT can trigger the "afterburn effect," where the body continues to burn calories even after the workout, further aiding in fat loss.

Benefits of Strength Training for Weight Loss

While cardio may be effective for burning calories, strength training, which includes exercises like weight lifting, resistance band workouts, and bodyweight exercises, has its own powerful benefits. Building lean muscle through strength training is especially valuable for long-term weight loss because muscle tissue burns more calories at rest than fat tissue. This increase in resting metabolic rate (RMR) can support ongoing fat loss, even when you're not actively exercising.

Strength training also contributes to body recomposition, allowing individuals to build muscle while losing fat, resulting in a toned appearance. In addition to aesthetic benefits, muscle strength improves functional fitness, making everyday tasks easier and helping prevent injuries. It also strengthens bones, which is especially important for older adults and those at risk of osteoporosis.

Cardio vs. Strength Training: Which is Better for Weight Loss?

For effective weight loss, a combination of both cardio and strength training is often the most beneficial approach. Cardio provides the calorie-burning advantage necessary to achieve a calorie deficit, while strength training promotes lean muscle growth and increases metabolism over time. This balance can lead to sustainable fat loss while preserving or even enhancing muscle tone.

Studies show that individuals who incorporate both types of exercise tend to have better long-term weight loss results compared to those who focus on only one form. For instance, pairing HIIT sessions with weightlifting can offer an optimal mix of calorie burn, muscle development, and cardiovascular health. Tailoring the balance of cardio and strength training to your specific goals and lifestyle can help you maintain consistency and enjoy your fitness journey.

How to Combine Cardio and Strength Training for Weight Loss

To maximize weight loss, aim for a blend of both cardio and strength sessions each week. Here's a sample weekly structure:

- **2–3 days of cardio** (including one HIIT session if desired) to enhance calorie burn and cardiovascular health.
- **2–3 days of strength training** focusing on all major muscle groups to build lean muscle and boost metabolism.
- **1 active recovery day** with activities like yoga or light walking to promote muscle recovery and reduce stress.

Listening to your body and adjusting your routine as you progress will ensure you avoid overtraining while achieving optimal results. With a balanced approach, cardio and strength training can work together to create a comprehensive fitness plan that supports weight loss and overall health.

Incorporating both cardio and strength training into your exercise routine can maximize fat loss, improve muscle tone, and promote long-term health. By finding the right mix that suits your goals and lifestyle, you'll set yourself up for lasting weight management and a stronger, healthier body.

The Science Behind High-Intensity Interval Training (HIIT)

High-Intensity Interval Training, or HIIT, has become one of the most popular and effective workouts for people aiming to lose weight, improve fitness, and increase overall health. HIIT involves alternating short bursts of intense exercise with periods of rest or lower-intensity movement. This style of workout leverages both aerobic and anaerobic systems, which helps burn calories quickly and boosts metabolism. The science behind HIIT supports its effectiveness for weight loss and cardiovascular health, making it a go-to for those looking for an efficient, time-saving workout.

How HIIT Burns Fat and Boosts Metabolism

One of the most impressive benefits of HIIT is its impact on fat burning and metabolic rate. During high-intensity intervals, your body works hard, often at 80–90% of your maximum heart rate, pushing it to burn calories at a rapid rate. After a HIIT workout, your metabolism stays elevated for hours due to a phenomenon known as Excess Post-Exercise Oxygen Consumption (EPOC), or the "afterburn effect." This means your body continues to burn calories even after you've stopped exercising, enhancing the overall calorie burn and aiding in fat loss.

HIIT also triggers changes at the cellular level, promoting increased mitochondrial activity. Mitochondria, often called the "powerhouses" of cells, help convert fuel into energy more efficiently. An increase in mitochondrial density improves the body's ability to burn fat, enhancing endurance and stamina over time.

Cardiovascular and Health Benefits of HIIT

In addition to weight loss, HIIT has substantial benefits for heart health. Studies have shown that it can help reduce blood pressure, regulate blood sugar, and improve cholesterol levels. HIIT workouts force your heart to work harder during intense bursts, which strengthens it over time and increases the amount of oxygen the body can consume in one exercise session, known as VO2 max. Improvements in VO2 max are linked with reduced risk of heart disease and better cardiovascular function, especially beneficial for those with sedentary lifestyles or early-stage heart concerns.

Moreover, HIIT may help improve insulin sensitivity, which is crucial for those at risk of type 2 diabetes. Improved insulin sensitivity allows the body to use glucose more effectively, decreasing the amount of glucose stored as fat.

HIIT for Busy Schedules: Maximizing Efficiency

HIIT's effectiveness is heightened by the fact that it can be completed in a shorter time frame than traditional workouts, making it ideal for those with tight schedules. A typical HIIT session can last from 10 to 30 minutes, yet it yields results comparable to, or even better than, longer, moderate-intensity workouts. Due to its efficiency, HIIT can be more sustainable than longer workouts for those who may struggle to find time for daily exercise. The variety of exercises—such as jumping jacks, sprints, and bodyweight exercises—keeps it engaging, making it easier to stick with long-term.

Conclusion

Exercise is a cornerstone of fat loss and overall health, providing benefits that go beyond what diet alone can achieve. By increasing metabolism, preserving muscle, enhancing cardiovascular health, and improving mental well-being, exercise lays the foundation for a healthier and more balanced life. When paired with nutritious eating, it creates a powerful approach to weight management that promotes long-lasting health and happiness.

Chapter 7

Building a Workout Routine That Fits Your Life

Creating a Balanced Fitness Plan: Cardio, Strength, Flexibility

Creating a balanced fitness plan is essential for improving overall health, increasing energy levels, and reaching specific fitness goals like weight loss, muscle gain, or enhanced flexibility. A comprehensive workout routine includes three main components: cardiovascular exercise (cardio), strength training, and flexibility exercises. Each element contributes unique benefits to physical well-being, and together, they form a well-rounded program that supports longevity, resilience, and functional fitness.

1. Cardiovascular Exercise (Cardio)

Cardio is any activity that raises your heart rate and gets your blood flowing, such as running, cycling, swimming, brisk walking, or dancing. Cardio is foundational to fitness because it strengthens the heart and lungs, improves circulation, and burns calories, aiding in weight management.

Benefits of Cardio

- **Heart Health:** Cardio strengthens the cardiovascular system, helping to lower blood pressure, improve blood flow, and reduce the risk of heart disease.
- **Weight Management:** Cardio burns calories, which can help create a calorie deficit necessary for weight loss.
- **Increased Stamina and Energy:** Regular cardio can improve endurance, making everyday tasks easier and enhancing overall energy levels.

- **Mental Health Boost:** Aerobic activities release endorphins, which boost mood and reduce symptoms of stress and anxiety.

Frequency and Types of Cardio

For a balanced routine, aim for at least 150 minutes of moderate-intensity cardio or 75 minutes of high-intensity cardio per week, as recommended by health experts. This could be broken down into 30 minutes a day, five days a week. Activities like running, brisk walking, swimming, and interval training are excellent choices. Mixing high-intensity workouts (e.g., sprinting or HIIT) with moderate activities (like walking or cycling) keeps the routine varied and sustainable.

2. Strength Training

Strength training, or resistance training, involves using weights, resistance bands, or body weight to work the muscles. Strength training is critical for building muscle mass, enhancing metabolism, and improving overall body composition.

Benefits of Strength Training

- **Increased Muscle Mass:** Builds and tones muscles, improving strength and aesthetic appearance.
- **Boosted Metabolism:** Muscles require more energy, even at rest, which can increase your resting metabolic rate and help with weight management.
- **Improved Bone Density:** Lifting weights places stress on bones, which can help increase bone density and lower the risk of osteoporosis.
- **Enhanced Functional Strength:** Strength training prepares the body for daily activities, reducing the risk of injury from routine tasks.

Frequency and Structure of Strength Training

Experts recommend performing strength training exercises at least two to three times a week, targeting all major muscle groups: legs, back, chest, shoulders, and core. Exercises like squats, lunges, push-ups, deadlifts, and rows are highly effective, as they engage multiple muscle groups. When beginning a strength training program, start with lighter weights and focus on form to avoid injury. Gradually increase the resistance as you become more comfortable and your muscles adapt.

3. Flexibility and Mobility Exercises

Flexibility exercises are often overlooked but are vital for maintaining joint health, preventing injuries, and enhancing performance in other types of exercise. Flexibility training includes static stretching, dynamic stretching, and yoga.

Benefits of Flexibility Training

- **Improved Range of Motion:** Stretching keeps muscles and joints flexible, allowing you to move more freely and reduce the risk of strains.
- **Enhanced Posture and Balance:** Flexibility exercises improve posture and balance by lengthening tight muscles, which can help prevent injuries.
- **Reduced Muscle Tension and Soreness:** Stretching can relieve muscle tension and help alleviate post-workout soreness.
- **Stress Relief:** Stretching exercises, like yoga, promote relaxation and reduce stress.

Types of Flexibility Exercises and Frequency

Incorporate flexibility exercises daily or at least three to four times a week, particularly after cardio or strength sessions, when muscles are warm. Dynamic stretches, like leg swings and arm circles, are ideal for warming up, while static stretches, like hamstring stretches or the child's pose, are better suited for cool downs. Yoga is also a highly effective practice, as it combines stretching, balance, and even strength, providing a holistic approach to flexibility.

Putting It All Together: Creating Your Balanced Plan

A well-rounded weekly plan may include the following:

- **Cardio:** 3–5 days a week, mixing moderate and high-intensity workouts.
- **Strength Training:** 2–3 days a week, focusing on different muscle groups each session.
- **Flexibility:** 3–5 days a week, with dynamic stretching before workouts and static stretching afterward.

For example:

- **Monday:** 30 minutes of moderate cardio (jogging or brisk walking) + flexibility (dynamic stretching)
- **Tuesday:** Strength training (upper body) + post-workout static stretching
- **Wednesday:** 20–30 minutes of HIIT cardio
- **Thursday:** Strength training (lower body) + post-workout static stretching
- **Friday:** Light cardio or rest day + flexibility (yoga session or stretching)
- **Saturday:** Full-body strength training + flexibility session
- **Sunday:** Rest day or low-intensity activity like a long walk or gentle stretching

Conclusion

Creating a balanced fitness plan with cardio, strength, and flexibility not only enhances overall health and wellness but also provides the versatility and resilience to adapt to life's demands.

With a blend of cardiovascular endurance, muscular strength, and flexibility, you'll be better equipped to achieve your fitness goals while preventing injuries and improving your quality of life. Adopting a balanced approach to fitness can lead to sustainable progress, enjoyable workouts, and a stronger, healthier body for years to come.

How to Stay Consistent and Make Exercise a Habit

Staying consistent with exercise and making it a habit can be a challenging endeavor, especially with a busy schedule or fluctuating motivation. However, establishing exercise as a lasting part of your life brings invaluable benefits, from improved physical health to better mental well-being. By focusing on practical strategies, setting achievable goals, and building a supportive environment, you can develop a consistent workout routine that fits seamlessly into your daily life.

1. Set Realistic Goals and Celebrate Progress

A common obstacle to staying consistent is setting unrealistic goals that quickly lead to burnout. Instead, aim to start small and celebrate every milestone along the way. Begin by defining what you want to achieve, such as improved strength, weight loss, or increased flexibility. Then break these larger goals down into manageable, short-term targets, like exercising three times a week for 30 minutes or walking 10,000 steps each day.

As you reach these smaller goals, celebrate your progress—whether it's lifting heavier weights, completing a full workout, or feeling more energized. Recognizing achievements, no matter how minor they seem, reinforces positive behaviors, making you more likely to continue.

2. Find Workouts You Enjoy

Exercise should be enjoyable, not a chore. By finding activities you genuinely like, you'll naturally look forward to your workouts. Experiment with different types of exercises, such as jogging, weight lifting, yoga, dancing, or group sports, until you find one or a few that keep you engaged. Trying new classes or activities can also bring variety to your routine, preventing boredom and making it easier to stay motivated. If traditional workouts don't appeal to you, look for creative ways to stay active, like hiking, swimming, or even gardening.

3. Schedule Workouts Like Appointments

Treating your workout like an essential meeting can help solidify exercise as a priority. Dedicate specific days and times for your workouts and add them to your calendar or planner. By carving out time in advance, you'll be less likely to skip a session or let other activities interfere. Mornings are often ideal for many people, as it's easier to stick to a routine before the day gets busy. However, if you're not a morning person, find a time that suits you best, whether it's during your lunch break or in the evening.

4. Create a Supportive Environment

Building an environment that promotes exercise makes it easier to stay consistent. Start by ensuring your workout gear is accessible and convenient. Lay out your exercise clothes the night before or keep them in your car or bag if you plan to work out after work. If you exercise at home, set up a designated area where you can work out comfortably, equipped with any tools or equipment you need.

Additionally, enlisting a workout buddy or joining a class can add accountability. Exercising with others creates a support system, making workouts more enjoyable and providing an extra push on days when motivation is low. Sharing goals with family or friends can also increase your commitment and help you stay consistent.

5. Overcome Obstacles with Backup Plans

Unplanned events, busy days, or fatigue can make it challenging to stick to your exercise plan. Creating backup options helps you stay active even when things don't go as planned. For example:

- **Shorter Workouts:** If you don't have time for a full session, fit in a quick 15-20 minute routine, such as bodyweight exercises or a brisk walk.
- **At-Home Options:** If you can't make it to the gym, have a few home workout videos or apps ready.
- **Bodyweight Exercises:** No equipment? Bodyweight exercises like squats, push-ups, and planks are convenient and effective.

These alternatives reduce the likelihood of skipping your workout altogether, allowing you to stay consistent despite challenges.

6. Track Your Progress and Adapt

Recording your progress provides a clear picture of your achievements and areas where you might need adjustments. Keep a journal or use an app to log your workouts, noting exercises, durations, or weights used. You can also track how you feel before and after workouts, which can help you recognize positive changes in mood or energy levels. Over time, reviewing your records can boost motivation and remind you of how far you've come.

Consistency doesn't mean doing the same thing every day—adapting your routine as your body grows stronger or as your goals shift is key. By modifying your workouts to challenge yourself appropriately, you prevent boredom and burnout, keeping the routine engaging and rewarding.

7. Emphasize Rest and Recovery

Rest days are an essential part of staying consistent. Allowing your body to recover helps prevent injury, reduces muscle soreness, and prepares you for your next workout. Rest doesn't have to mean complete inactivity; consider incorporating active recovery, like light stretching, a gentle walk, or yoga. These low-intensity activities help relieve tension, boost circulation, and keep you engaged with the habit of staying active.

8. Make Exercise Part of Your Identity

One of the most powerful strategies for building a lasting habit is to see yourself as someone who values fitness. Instead of viewing exercise as an external obligation, think of it as part of who you are. Each time you make a choice to prioritize your health—whether by completing a workout, choosing healthier foods, or staying active—you reinforce this identity. Over time, your consistent actions will help solidify a self-image centered on wellness, making exercise a natural part of your life.

Adapting Workouts for Home, Gym, or Outdoor Settings

Creating a workout routine that suits your lifestyle means being able to adapt to different settings—whether you're at home, in a gym, or enjoying the outdoors. Each setting offers unique benefits and challenges, and with some flexibility and creativity, you can get an effective workout no matter where you are. Here's how to tailor your fitness routine to fit each environment, ensuring you stay consistent and motivated.

1. Home Workouts

Advantages: Home workouts are convenient, budget-friendly, and provide privacy, allowing you to exercise comfortably without time spent commuting. Home also allows for flexibility, making it easier to incorporate short workouts throughout the day.

Equipment: You don't need a fully stocked gym at home to build a complete fitness routine. Simple, versatile equipment like resistance bands, dumbbells, a jump rope, or a yoga mat can go a long way. Bodyweight exercises (e.g., push-ups, squats, lunges, and planks) are also incredibly effective for building strength and cardiovascular fitness.

Types of Workouts:

- **Strength Training**: Use dumbbells, kettlebells, or body weight for strength exercises. Circuit-style strength training, where you move quickly from one exercise to the next, is ideal for efficient muscle-building.
- **Cardio**: Jump rope, high-intensity interval training (HIIT), or even dancing in your living room can provide a great cardio workout.
- **Flexibility and Mobility**: Incorporate yoga or stretching sessions that don't require any equipment. These can also double as relaxation exercises and stress relief.

Tips for Success:

- Dedicate a specific area in your home for workouts, even if it's just a corner with enough space to move comfortably.
- Establish a routine to create consistency, such as working out first thing in the morning or during lunch breaks.
- Find virtual classes or follow online trainers for guidance and motivation if you're unsure where to start.

2. Gym Workouts

Advantages: The gym provides access to a wide range of equipment, trainers, and amenities, which can help enhance the variety and effectiveness of your workouts. For those who enjoy the social aspect of fitness, gyms also offer group classes and the chance to meet others with similar goals.

Equipment: Gyms have all the tools you might need, from free weights to cardio machines to specialized equipment like rowing machines and cable stations. This allows you to perform a range of exercises that might not be feasible at home.

Types of Workouts:

- **Strength Training**: Use free weights, resistance machines, and cable machines for targeted strength exercises. Training different muscle groups on different days, known as split routines, is popular for maximizing muscle growth and recovery.
- **Cardio**: Treadmills, ellipticals, rowing machines, and stationary bikes provide various options for cardio workouts, and most machines can be adjusted for your fitness level.
- **Flexibility and Mobility**: Many gyms offer yoga and stretching areas where you can work on flexibility. Some even provide foam rollers for muscle recovery.

Tips for Success:

- Create a plan before you arrive to stay focused and avoid wasting time.
- Consider working with a personal trainer to learn proper techniques and build a personalized plan.
- If you find the gym intimidating, try quieter hours or group classes that can make the environment more welcoming.

3. Outdoor Workouts

Advantages: Exercising outdoors is refreshing, cost-free, and has proven mental health benefits, such as stress reduction and improved mood. Nature provides varied terrain, which can be an added challenge and help improve functional fitness.

Equipment: While outdoor workouts often require minimal equipment, items like a yoga mat, resistance bands, or even a kettlebell can add variety. Many parks and trails also have built-in fitness stations, pull-up bars, or stairs that can be used creatively in a workout.

Types of Workouts:

- **Cardio**: Running, hiking, biking, or even brisk walking are excellent cardio options outdoors. Interval training can be incorporated by alternating jogging with sprints.
- **Strength Training**: Use benches, walls, or monkey bars in playgrounds for bodyweight exercises like dips, pull-ups, and incline push-ups.
- **Flexibility and Mobility**: Find a quiet, flat space for yoga or stretching. Outdoor yoga sessions provide an added benefit of connecting with nature, enhancing relaxation and focus.

Tips for Success:

- Choose safe, well-lit areas and be mindful of weather conditions.
- Use trails, stairs, and hills for natural resistance and variety.
- Wear appropriate gear, like supportive shoes and weather-appropriate clothing, to make outdoor workouts comfortable.

Final Thoughts

Creating a consistent exercise habit isn't about perfection; it's about finding a sustainable approach that fits your lifestyle. By setting realistic goals, finding enjoyable workouts, scheduling sessions, building a supportive environment, and remaining adaptable, you can make exercise a regular part of your life. Remember that setbacks are natural, and it's more important to stay committed to the journey than to strive for flawless execution. Embracing exercise as part of your identity and lifestyle will set you up for long-term success, bringing you the benefits of physical fitness, mental resilience, and overall well-being.

Adapting workouts to different settings not only keeps your routine interesting but also builds your ability to stay consistent regardless of circumstances. Home workouts, gym sessions, and outdoor exercises all offer unique benefits that, when combined, can provide a well-rounded approach to fitness. By making the most of each environment and incorporating elements of cardio, strength, and flexibility, you're setting up a balanced, versatile routine that can fit seamlessly into your life.

Chapter 8

Strength Training for Fat Loss and Muscle Building

Lifting Weights to Lose Weight: The Benefits of Strength Training

Strength training is often overlooked in weight loss discussions, with cardio exercises like running or cycling taking the spotlight. However, lifting weights is one of the most effective methods for not only losing weight but also reshaping and strengthening the body. Here's an in-depth look at how strength training contributes to fat loss, boosts metabolism, and supports sustainable weight management.

1. Boosts Metabolic Rate

Strength training increases your resting metabolic rate (RMR), which means your body burns more calories even when you're not actively exercising. Unlike cardio, where calorie burn typically stops after the workout, strength training creates a longer-lasting impact through a phenomenon known as *excess post-exercise oxygen consumption* (EPOC). Following a strength workout, your body continues to burn calories at an elevated rate for up to 48 hours. This effect, also called the "afterburn," means that the more muscle you build, the more efficiently your body burns calories around the clock.

2. Preserves and Builds Lean Muscle Mass

One of the challenges in weight loss is avoiding the loss of lean muscle mass. Cardio-heavy weight loss routines often lead to muscle loss along with fat loss, which can lower metabolism over time. Strength training helps counter this by promoting muscle growth, which helps your body retain lean mass even as you lose fat. Muscle tissue is more metabolically active than fat, meaning it requires more energy to maintain. By building muscle, you create a body composition that supports ongoing fat loss.

3. Increases Fat-Burning Potential

Strength training helps your body target fat for energy instead of muscle. This approach leads to a higher proportion of fat loss rather than simply weight loss, making your weight loss results more sustainable. Additionally, with more lean muscle, your body is better equipped to handle higher-intensity exercises, allowing you to incorporate more demanding workouts as you progress, further enhancing fat-burning potential.

4. Improves Body Composition and Tone

While cardio often results in a slimmer physique, strength training changes the composition of your body by reducing fat and increasing muscle definition. This combination leads to a toned and firm appearance. Even at a similar weight, someone who incorporates strength training into their routine may appear leaner and more defined due to the higher muscle-to-fat ratio. By focusing on strength training, you can achieve a body composition that feels both strong and healthy.

5. Supports Better Mental Health and Stress Management

Lifting weights has mental health benefits as well, which indirectly supports weight loss. Strength training can reduce stress, enhance mood, and improve sleep quality, all of which are essential for maintaining a balanced lifestyle. Exercise, especially strength-focused workouts, stimulates the release of endorphins, which improve mood and provide a natural boost of energy. Better mental health and lower stress levels can reduce the urge for emotional eating, leading to healthier, more mindful choices.

6. Supports Long-Term Weight Maintenance

Unlike extreme diets or cardio-heavy plans that may yield short-term results, strength training fosters long-term weight loss by creating a body that efficiently burns calories and supports a stable metabolic rate. This means that even after reaching your weight goal, strength training helps you maintain it by preventing the common pitfall of regaining weight. Consistent strength training fosters a lifestyle that supports healthy weight management.

7. Enhances Everyday Functionality and Mobility

Strength training isn't just about losing weight; it's also about improving daily functional movements. By strengthening muscles, joints, and bones, you'll improve mobility, posture, and balance, which can prevent injuries and enhance overall quality of life. As we age, muscle mass naturally decreases, but strength training can counteract this decline, helping you stay active, agile, and independent.

8. Flexible Options for All Fitness Levels

The beauty of strength training is its adaptability; it can be customized for any fitness level. Beginners can start with bodyweight exercises or resistance bands, while more experienced individuals might use free weights or machines. Strength training can be performed anywhere, whether at the gym, at home, or outside, making it accessible and easy to fit into any lifestyle.

Key Strength Training Exercises for Every Fitness Level

Strength training doesn't require extreme lifting or advanced moves to be effective. For weight loss, muscle building, and overall health, mastering a few fundamental exercises is essential. These exercises can be adjusted for beginners, intermediate, and advanced fitness levels, making them adaptable and versatile as you progress. Here's a breakdown of essential strength training exercises that cater to all fitness levels, their benefits, and variations to suit your journey.

1. Squats

Benefits: Squats are a full-body exercise that primarily targets the lower body muscles, including the quads, glutes, hamstrings, and calves, while engaging the core. They build leg strength, enhance functional mobility, and support fat burning.

Variations for Different Levels:

- **Beginner: Bodyweight Squat** – Start by doing squats with just your body weight. Focus on form, ensuring that your knees don't go past your toes and your back remains straight.
- **Intermediate: Goblet Squat** – Hold a dumbbell or kettlebell close to your chest to add resistance, which will increase strength in your legs and core.
- **Advanced: Barbell Back Squat** – Add a barbell on your upper back. This version allows for increased weight, which intensifies strength building in the legs and glutes.

2. Push-Ups

Benefits: Push-ups target the chest, shoulders, triceps, and core. They are excellent for building upper body strength and endurance while engaging multiple muscle groups.

Variations for Different Levels:

- **Beginner: Incline Push-Up** – Place your hands on a higher surface like a bench or countertop. This reduces the intensity but allows you to build foundational strength.
- **Intermediate: Standard Push-Up** – Perform push-ups on the floor with your body in a straight line, engaging your core.
- **Advanced: Decline Push-Up** – Elevate your feet on a bench or step, making the exercise more challenging for the upper chest and shoulders.

3. Lunges

Benefits: Lunges are a compound exercise that works the glutes, quads, hamstrings, and calves. They also help improve balance and core stability.

Variations for Different Levels:

- **Beginner: Stationary Lunge** – Start by doing a static lunge without stepping forward. Focus on balance and control.
- **Intermediate: Walking Lunge** – Step forward with each lunge, alternating legs. This version builds stability and strength.
- **Advanced: Weighted Reverse Lunge** – Hold a dumbbell in each hand while performing a reverse lunge, which increases intensity and engages the core further.

4. Deadlifts

Benefits: Deadlifts strengthen the hamstrings, glutes, lower back, and core. They're effective for building overall power and improving posture.

Variations for Different Levels:

- **Beginner: Dumbbell Romanian Deadlift** – Use light dumbbells to practice form and strengthen the posterior chain (back of the body).
- **Intermediate: Barbell Deadlift** – With a barbell, increase the weight to engage the glutes, hamstrings, and lower back more intensively.
- **Advanced: Single-Leg Deadlift** – Perform the exercise on one leg, holding a dumbbell or kettlebell, which adds difficulty and challenges balance.

5. Planks

Benefits: Planks are an isometric exercise that builds core strength and stability. They work the abs, obliques, lower back, and shoulders.

Variations for Different Levels:

- **Beginner: Knee Plank** – Start by holding a plank position on your knees, which reduces the intensity but helps build core strength.
- **Intermediate: Standard Plank** – Hold a straight plank position on your toes, ensuring your back remains flat and your core engaged.
- **Advanced: Side Plank** – Try side planks for extra core engagement, particularly in the obliques. Add leg lifts or arm reaches to increase the challenge.

6. Rows

Benefits: Rows target the back muscles, including the lats, rhomboids, and traps, and are crucial for upper body strength and posture improvement.

Variations for Different Levels:

- **Beginner: Seated Cable Row** – Use a cable machine to perform seated rows, focusing on pulling from the back rather than the arms.
- **Intermediate: Bent-Over Dumbbell Row** – With a slight bend in the knees, hinge at the waist and row dumbbells toward your hips, keeping the back straight.
- **Advanced: Barbell Row** – Use a barbell with increased weight, keeping your core tight and focusing on pulling the bar toward your lower ribs.

7. Shoulder Press

Benefits: The shoulder press builds strength in the shoulders, upper chest, and triceps. It's a foundational exercise for upper body strength and stability.

Variations for Different Levels:

- **Beginner: Seated Dumbbell Shoulder Press** – Sit on a bench and use light dumbbells, focusing on controlled movements.
- **Intermediate: Standing Dumbbell Shoulder Press** – Stand while pressing the dumbbells overhead, which engages the core and improves stability.
- **Advanced: Barbell Shoulder Press** – Use a barbell with increased weight to challenge the shoulders and upper chest further.

8. Glute Bridges or Hip Thrusts

Benefits: These exercises target the glutes, hamstrings, and lower back, improving strength and stability in the lower body.

Variations for Different Levels:

- **Beginner: Bodyweight Glute Bridge** – Lie on your back with knees bent and lift your hips toward the ceiling, focusing on glute activation.
- **Intermediate: Single-Leg Glute Bridge** – Lift one leg off the ground and perform the bridge with the other leg for added difficulty.
- **Advanced: Barbell Hip Thrust** – Place a barbell across your hips and thrust up, engaging the glutes and increasing resistance.

Progress Tracking: How to Increase Strength and Keep Results Coming

Tracking progress is a powerful tool in strength training, helping you stay motivated, pinpoint areas for improvement, and celebrate milestones. A well-structured progress tracking plan provides insights into your growth and guides how to make adjustments to keep seeing results. Here's how to effectively track progress, set realistic goals, and adapt your routine to continuously increase strength and stay on course.

1. Set Clear, Measurable Goals

Before starting, identify specific, achievable goals that align with your larger fitness objectives. Examples include increasing the weight you can deadlift, improving your push-up count, or hitting a target number of reps for a specific exercise. These goals give your training sessions direction and give you something concrete to work toward.

Tips for Setting Strength Goals:

- **Break Down Larger Goals**: If your goal is to deadlift 200 pounds, set smaller incremental goals like 150, 175, and finally 200 pounds. This keeps your progress manageable and easier to track.
- **Establish a Timeline**: Create a timeframe, like aiming for an increase within 12 weeks, to add focus and urgency.
- **Keep It Realistic**: Gradual progress builds sustainable strength, so avoid overloading too quickly.

2. Use a Training Log

A training log or workout journal helps you track every workout, noting weights, reps, sets, and rest periods. Recording each detail allows you to observe trends over time, identify plateaus, and adjust as needed. Many people use notebooks, spreadsheets, or apps dedicated to fitness tracking.

What to Record:

- **Weight and Sets/Reps**: Note the weight used for each exercise and the number of sets and reps completed. Tracking this for every session allows you to see if you're lifting heavier over time.
- **Exercise Order**: Tracking the sequence of exercises can help you see if you're improving in specific movements.
- **Additional Notes**: Make a note of how you felt during the workout—e.g., if you were sore, tired, or energized. This helps correlate performance with factors like rest, hydration, or nutrition.

3. Progressive Overload: The Key to Continuous Improvement

Progressive overload is the principle of gradually increasing the stress placed on your muscles during workouts. By consistently challenging your muscles with heavier weights, more reps, or different variations, you encourage growth and strength development. Implementing progressive overload is crucial for breaking through plateaus and continuing to see improvements.

Methods of Progressive Overload:

- **Increase Weight**: Lifting heavier weights is the most direct way to apply overload. Try to increase by small increments, such as 2.5-5 pounds, each week or every few weeks.
- **Add Reps or Sets**: If you're not ready to increase weight, try doing more reps or adding an extra set to your routine.
- **Decrease Rest Time**: Shortening rest periods between sets places greater demand on your muscles, pushing them to adapt.

- **Change Tempo**: Slow down your movements or pause at specific points in the exercise. This intensifies muscle engagement without necessarily increasing weight.

4. Use Strength Testing Benchmarks

Strength tests are checkpoints to gauge your performance over time. Set specific intervals—such as every 4-6 weeks—for these assessments to measure your progress and adjust your goals as needed. These benchmarks can range from lifting a certain weight to completing bodyweight exercises within a time frame.

Popular Strength Benchmarks:

- **1-Rep Max (1RM)**: Test the maximum weight you can lift for one rep. Commonly used for exercises like the bench press, squat, and deadlift, the 1RM measures peak strength.
- **AMRAP (As Many Reps As Possible)**: Set a weight you're comfortable with and perform as many reps as possible before reaching failure. This is an excellent way to gauge endurance.
- **Timed Holds**: Exercises like planks or wall sits can be timed to see how long you can hold the position, which is a great measure of endurance and stability.

5. Take Progress Photos and Body Measurements

While strength metrics are essential, photos and measurements offer a visual and physical representation of your progress, especially if fat loss or muscle definition is part of your goal. Taking progress photos at regular intervals (e.g., every month) and measuring key areas (arms, chest, waist, hips, thighs) give you more ways to see changes over time.

Tips for Effective Progress Tracking:

- **Use Consistent Angles**: Take front, side, and back photos under the same lighting conditions for better comparison.
- **Measure at the Same Time**: Ideally, do measurements in the morning to avoid inconsistencies due to daily fluctuations.
- **Avoid Over-Measuring**: Stick to monthly intervals for photos and measurements to avoid discouragement from natural body changes.

6. Incorporate Periodization for Long-Term Success

Periodization is the strategy of dividing your training into different phases, such as strength, hypertrophy (muscle building), and endurance. Cycling through these phases prevents your body from adapting to the same routine, which can slow progress. Periodization ensures your muscles are consistently challenged and helps maintain motivation by adding variety.

Example of a Simple Periodization Cycle:

- **Weeks 1-4 (Strength Focus)**: Lower reps (3-5 per set) with higher weights to build strength.
- **Weeks 5-8 (Hypertrophy Focus)**: Moderate reps (8-12 per set) with slightly lower weight for muscle growth.
- **Weeks 9-12 (Endurance Focus)**: Higher reps (12-15 per set) with lighter weights to build muscle endurance.

7. Celebrate and Adjust Based on Progress

Strength training is a long-term commitment, and each small success deserves recognition. Tracking milestones like hitting a new weight target or mastering a challenging move keeps motivation high. If you hit a plateau, evaluate your routine and make adjustments to keep progressing. Sometimes this means shifting focus from one exercise to another, adjusting rep schemes, or even taking a short recovery phase.

Key Points to Re-Evaluate When Progress Stalls:

- **Recovery**: Ensure you're allowing enough rest for muscles to repair and grow.
- **Nutrition**: A diet rich in protein and adequate calories supports muscle building and strength.
- **Routine Variation**: Changing exercises or introducing new methods like supersets can help re-engage your muscles.

Final Thoughts

Strength training offers comprehensive benefits for those looking to lose weight and keep it off. By boosting metabolism, preserving muscle, and reshaping the body, strength training provides a sustainable path to weight loss. Its impact extends beyond weight loss, promoting better mental health, increased functionality, and lasting physical well-being. For those embarking on a weight loss journey, adding strength training to your routine could be the key to achieving a healthier, stronger, and leaner body that supports long-term goals.

No matter your fitness level, these exercises provide a comprehensive foundation for strength training. Each one can be adapted to meet your current abilities and scaled up as you progress. By incorporating these moves into your routine, you'll build strength, improve muscle tone, and support fat loss with a balanced approach. Embrace each level, focus on proper form, and enjoy the journey toward a stronger, healthier body.

Tracking your progress and consistently aiming for improvement is essential in a successful strength training journey. Setting clear goals, progressively challenging yourself, and using benchmarks allow you to assess your growth, make necessary adjustments, and continue to see results. Strength training is not about instant changes but steady progress. Celebrate every achievement, big or small, and remember that each effort adds up to long-term success in fitness and health.

Chapter 9

Effective Cardio Workouts for Fat Burn

<u>Best Cardio Workouts for Maximum Fat Burn</u>

Cardio workouts are an essential component of any fat loss program. They elevate your heart rate, increase calorie burn, and boost your metabolism, helping your body tap into fat stores for energy. However, not all cardio workouts are created equal when it comes to maximizing fat burn. Choosing the right type of cardio and tailoring it to your fitness level and goals can make a significant difference. Here's a detailed look at the best cardio workouts for effective fat burning.

1. High-Intensity Interval Training (HIIT)

Why It Works: HIIT alternates between short bursts of intense activity and periods of lower intensity or rest. This method not only burns a high number of calories in a short amount of time but also boosts your metabolism for hours after your workout, a phenomenon known as **excess post-exercise oxygen consumption (EPOC).**

Benefits:

- Burns fat while preserving muscle mass.
- Increases cardiovascular endurance.
- Can be done in as little as 20-30 minutes.

Examples:

- **Sprints:** 30 seconds of sprinting followed by 1-2 minutes of walking or jogging, repeated for 20 minutes.
- **Cycling:** 20 seconds of all-out pedaling followed by 40 seconds of slow cycling.

- **Bodyweight HIIT:** Jump squats, burpees, and mountain climbers for 30 seconds each, with 15-second rest periods.

2. Steady-State Cardio

Why It Works: Steady-state cardio involves maintaining a consistent pace and intensity over an extended period. While it doesn't burn as many calories per minute as HIIT, it's excellent for improving endurance and burning fat, especially when performed in the **fat-burning zone** (about 60-70% of your maximum heart rate).

Benefits:

- Easier on the joints and muscles.
- Suitable for beginners or as an active recovery workout.
- Can be sustained for longer durations, increasing total calorie burn.

Examples:

- **Brisk Walking or Light Jogging:** 30-60 minutes at a moderate pace.
- **Cycling at a Steady Pace:** 45-60 minutes on a flat or moderately hilly route.
- **Swimming:** Continuous laps for 30-45 minutes.

3. Circuit Training with Cardio Moves

Why It Works: Circuit training combines strength exercises with cardio bursts, such as jumping jacks or jump rope. This keeps your heart rate elevated while building muscle, offering a dual benefit of fat burn and muscle development.

Benefits:

- Increases calorie burn by combining strength and cardio.
- Improves overall fitness and body composition.

- Provides variety, making workouts more engaging.

Examples:

- Perform a circuit of squats, push-ups, and lunges, interspersed with 1-minute intervals of high knees or jumping rope.
- Kettlebell swings followed by a 1-minute sprint.

4. Running and Incline Training

Why It Works: Running, particularly on an incline, requires more effort and engages larger muscle groups, resulting in a higher calorie burn. Treadmill users can increase the incline, while outdoor runners can choose hilly routes.

Benefits:

- Highly effective for burning calories in a short period.
- Builds lower body strength and endurance.
- Can be easily adjusted to match fitness levels.

Examples:

- **Hill Sprints:** Sprint uphill for 20-30 seconds, then walk back down for recovery.
- **Incline Treadmill Walking:** Set the incline to 10-15% and walk briskly for 30 minutes.

5. Rowing

Why It Works: Rowing provides a full-body workout, engaging both upper and lower body muscles. It's an excellent way to burn calories and fat while improving strength and cardiovascular fitness.

Benefits:

- Works 85% of the body's muscles.
- Low impact, making it joint-friendly.
- Can be performed at varying intensities.

Examples:

- Perform steady-state rowing for 30 minutes.
- Alternate 1 minute of high-intensity rowing with 2 minutes of moderate rowing for a HIIT-style workout.

6. Jump Rope

Why It Works: Jumping rope is an efficient cardio exercise that burns a significant number of calories in a short amount of time. It also improves coordination, agility, and cardiovascular endurance.

Benefits:

- Portable and inexpensive.
- Can burn up to 10 calories per minute.
- Improves overall cardiovascular health.

Examples:

- Jump for 1 minute at a moderate pace, then rest for 30 seconds. Repeat for 15-20 minutes.
- Combine jump rope intervals with bodyweight exercises like push-ups or squats.

7. Swimming

Why It Works: Swimming engages the entire body while providing a low-impact workout. It's especially effective for those with joint issues or injuries, as it reduces stress on the body while still delivering a high calorie burn.

Benefits:

- Full-body workout with minimal joint strain.
- Improves cardiovascular health and builds endurance.
- Can be adapted for all fitness levels.

Examples:

- Swim laps at a moderate pace for 30-45 minutes.
- Alternate between slow and fast laps for a HIIT-style swim workout.

Low-Impact vs. High-Impact Cardio: Which is Best for You?

When it comes to cardio workouts, you often hear about **low-impact** and **high-impact** exercises. Both types have their benefits and drawbacks, and understanding which one suits your fitness level, goals, and physical condition can help you design an effective and sustainable workout routine. This guide will explore the differences between low-impact and high-impact cardio, their benefits, and how to choose the best option for your needs.

Understanding Low-Impact Cardio

Definition:
Low-impact cardio exercises involve movements where at least one foot stays in contact with the ground at all times, or the exercise minimizes joint stress. These workouts are gentle on the joints and ideal for beginners, those recovering from injuries, or individuals with chronic joint pain.

Examples:

- Walking
- Cycling
- Swimming
- Rowing
- Elliptical machine workouts
- Yoga and Pilates (when focused on cardio)

Benefits of Low-Impact Cardio:

1. **Joint-Friendly:** Low-impact exercises reduce stress on the knees, hips, and ankles, making them ideal for people with joint issues or arthritis.
2. **Accessible for All Fitness Levels:** These workouts are suitable for beginners, older adults, or those returning to exercise after a break.

3. **Supports Recovery:** Low-impact exercises are excellent for active recovery days as they keep you moving without overloading your body.
4. **Improves Cardiovascular Health:** Regular low-impact cardio can enhance heart health, improve endurance, and aid in fat loss.

Understanding High-Impact Cardio

Definition:
High-impact cardio exercises involve movements where both feet leave the ground simultaneously at certain points, or the exercises exert more force on your joints. These workouts typically burn more calories and build explosive strength but require a higher level of fitness and joint stability.

Examples:

- Running or jogging
- Jumping jacks
- Burpees
- Plyometric exercises (e.g., jump squats, box jumps)
- High-intensity interval training (HIIT)
- Dance workouts like Zumba

Benefits of High-Impact Cardio:

1. **Higher Calorie Burn:** These workouts elevate your heart rate quickly, leading to more calories burned in a shorter period.
2. **Builds Bone Density:** The impact from exercises like running or jumping helps stimulate bone growth and prevent osteoporosis.
3. **Enhances Athletic Performance:** High-impact exercises improve agility, coordination, and explosive power, benefiting those engaged in sports or performance training.

4. **Boosts Metabolic Rate:** High-impact cardio often leads to greater post-exercise calorie burn due to **excess post-exercise oxygen consumption (EPOC).**

Key Differences between Low-Impact and High-Impact Cardio

Aspect	Low-Impact Cardio	High-Impact Cardio
Joint Stress	Minimal	High
Calorie Burn Rate	Moderate	High
Suitability	Best for beginners, recovery, or joint issues	Best for advanced fitness levels or performance goals
Bone Health Benefits	Minimal	High
Cardiovascular Impact	Improves endurance over time	Quick improvement in heart rate and stamina
Injury Risk	Low	Higher, especially without proper form or warm-up

How to Choose the Best Option for You

1. **Assess Your Fitness Level:** If you're just starting your fitness journey or recovering from an injury, low-impact exercises are a great way to build endurance without overwhelming your body. Advanced individuals looking for a challenge might prefer high-impact workouts for faster results.
2. **Consider Your Goals:**
   - If your goal is **fat loss**, both types can be effective. High-impact workouts typically burn more calories, but low-impact options are sustainable for longer durations.
   - If you're aiming for **improved cardiovascular health**, consistency is key. Choose the type of exercise that you'll enjoy and stick with over time.
   - For **bone health**, incorporate high-impact cardio if your body can handle it.
3. **Listen to Your Body:** Joint pain or discomfort during or after high-impact exercises may indicate the need to switch to low-impact options. Conversely, if low-impact workouts feel too easy, gradually incorporate high-impact moves.
4. **Mix It Up:** A combination of both low-impact and high-impact exercises can offer the best of both worlds. This approach can prevent workout monotony, reduce injury risk, and target different aspects of fitness.

Sample Workout Plans

Low-Impact Cardio Routine (30-45 Minutes):

- 10 minutes: Warm-up with brisk walking or cycling.
- 20 minutes: Moderate-intensity swimming or elliptical training.
- 10-15 minutes: Cool down with light stretching or yoga.

High-Impact Cardio Routine (20-30 Minutes):

- 5 minutes: Dynamic warm-up (e.g., jumping jacks, light jogging).
- 15-20 minutes: HIIT (e.g., 30 seconds of burpees, 1-minute rest, repeat).
- 5 minutes: Cool down with static stretching.

How to Incorporate Fun Cardio Like Dance, Sports, or Hiking

Cardio doesn't have to be monotonous or confined to treadmills and stationary bikes. One of the best ways to make cardiovascular exercise enjoyable and sustainable is by engaging in activities that are not only effective for fat burning but also fun and engaging. Dance, sports, and hiking are excellent examples of activities that combine physical exertion with enjoyment, making it easier to stick to your fitness goals. Here's how you can incorporate these activities into your routine to maximize fat burn while having a great time.

The Benefits of Fun Cardio Activities

1. **Increased Motivation:** Fun activities like dancing or playing sports are less likely to feel like a chore, which keeps you motivated to stay consistent.
2. **High-Calorie Burn:** Many of these activities are high-intensity and can burn a significant amount of calories, aiding in fat loss.
3. **Improved Mental Health:** Engaging in enjoyable cardio can reduce stress, improve mood, and combat anxiety, thanks to the release of endorphins.
4. **Social Interaction:** Activities like team sports and group dance classes offer social opportunities, which can boost accountability and make workouts more enjoyable.

Dance for Cardio and Fat Burn

Why Dance? Dance is a dynamic cardio workout that improves cardiovascular health, enhances coordination, and burns calories. Whether it's a structured dance class or freestyle dancing at home, it's a fantastic way to stay active.

Types of Dance Workouts:

- **Zumba:** Combines Latin-inspired moves with high-energy music for a full-body workout.
- **Hip-Hop Dance:** Involves fast-paced, high-impact moves that can burn up to 500 calories per hour.
- **Ballet Barre:** Focuses on low-impact movements that improve flexibility and muscle endurance.
- **Freestyle Dancing:** Allows you to move freely to your favorite music, making it a flexible and personalized workout.

How to Incorporate Dance:

- Join a local dance class or sign up for online sessions.
- Dedicate 20-30 minutes to freestyle dancing at home to your favorite playlist.
- Incorporate dance breaks during your day for a quick energy boost.

Sports for an Engaging Cardio Routine

Why Sports? Playing sports combines cardio, strength, and agility training. The dynamic movements involved in sports help build endurance, improve coordination, and burn fat.

Popular Sports for Cardio:

- **Soccer:** Provides an intense workout with sprints, endurance runs, and dynamic movements.
- **Basketball:** Combines running, jumping, and agility drills, burning up to 600 calories per hour.
- **Tennis:** Involves quick lateral movements and bursts of running, making it a great cardio option.
- **Ultimate Frisbee:** Offers a full-body workout with running, jumping, and throwing.

How to Incorporate Sports:

- Join a local league or recreational team.
- Schedule weekly pick-up games with friends or coworkers.
- Use sports as a weekend activity to replace traditional workouts.

Hiking: A Natural Cardio Workout

Why Hiking? Hiking is a low-impact yet highly effective cardio workout that builds endurance and strengthens lower-body muscles. It's also an excellent way to connect with nature, which can improve mental clarity and reduce stress.

Benefits of Hiking for Cardio:

- **Variable Intensity:** Uphill climbs and varied terrain increase heart rate and calorie burn.
- **Full-Body Engagement:** Incorporates muscles in the legs, core, and sometimes the upper body when using trekking poles.
- **Mental Health Boost:** Time in nature has been shown to reduce stress and improve mood.

How to Incorporate Hiking:

- Start with local trails and gradually progress to more challenging terrains.
- Aim for one hike per week as part of your cardio routine.
- Combine hiking with other outdoor activities like camping for a full weekend of physical activity.

Combining Fun Cardio with Your Fitness Goals

1. **Set a Schedule:** Treat your fun cardio sessions like any other workout by scheduling them into your week. Aim for at least 150 minutes of moderate or 75 minutes of vigorous activity weekly.

2. **Mix It Up:** Keep things fresh by alternating between different activities. For example, you could dance on Mondays, play basketball on Wednesdays, and go hiking on Saturdays.
3. **Track Your Progress:** Use a fitness tracker or app to monitor your heart rate and calories burned during these activities. This can help you measure the effectiveness of your workouts and keep you motivated.
4. **Get Social:** Invite friends or family to join your activities. This adds a social element, increasing the likelihood of sticking to your routine.

Final Thoughts

The best cardio workout for fat burn depends on your fitness level, preferences, and goals. High-Intensity Interval Training (HIIT) offers maximum calorie burn in minimal time, while steady-state cardio provides a sustainable approach for those looking to build endurance. Whether you prefer running, swimming, or circuit training, the key is consistency and finding a workout style you enjoy. Combining different types of cardio can also keep your routine fresh and engaging, ensuring long-term success in your fat-burning journey.

Both low-impact and high-impact cardio offer unique benefits, and the best choice depends on your fitness level, goals, and physical condition. Whether you're looking to burn fat, improve heart health, or boost endurance, incorporating the right type of cardio into your routine can help you achieve sustainable results. Remember, the key to success is consistency, so choose exercises you enjoy and can perform regularly.

Incorporating fun cardio activities like dance, sports, and hiking can transform your workout routine from a chore into something you genuinely look forward to. These activities not only help you burn fat and improve cardiovascular health but also boost mental well-being and provide opportunities for social interaction. The key to long-term success is finding an activity you enjoy and making it a regular part of your lifestyle. Whether you're grooving to your favorite tunes, scoring goals on the field, or exploring scenic trails, fun cardio ensures you'll stay consistent while achieving your fitness goals.

Chapter 10

Staying Active in Everyday Life

How Small Activities Throughout the Day Can Help Burn Calories

When it comes to staying active and burning calories, every movement counts. You don't need a formal workout session to increase your daily energy expenditure. Small, seemingly insignificant activities, often referred to as **Non-Exercise Activity Thermogenesis (NEAT)**, can make a big difference in your overall calorie burn and contribute to weight management and better health. This concept focuses on staying active throughout the day, even outside of structured exercise, by integrating small bursts of movement into your daily routine.

What Is NEAT and Why Does It Matter?

NEAT refers to the energy expended during activities that aren't traditional exercise, like walking to your car, cleaning the house, or fidgeting at your desk. It includes everything from standing while working to playing with your kids. These activities may seem minor, but they can significantly contribute to your daily calorie burn.

Why NEAT Matters:

- Helps offset the effects of a sedentary lifestyle.
- Increases daily calorie expenditure without requiring intense workouts.
- Supports weight loss and maintenance.
- Improves overall health by reducing prolonged periods of inactivity.

Simple Activities That Boost Calorie Burn

Here are practical ways to incorporate small activities into your day and increase your NEAT:

1. Take the Stairs

Why It Helps: Climbing stairs engages your leg muscles and increases your heart rate, burning more calories than standing or taking the elevator. It's a simple yet effective way to add more movement to your day.

How to Incorporate:

- Choose stairs over elevators or escalators whenever possible.
- If you work in a multi-story building, challenge yourself to climb a few flights daily.

2. Walk More Frequently

Why It Helps: Walking is one of the easiest and most accessible ways to burn extra calories. Even short walks add up over time.

How to Incorporate:

- Park farther from the entrance when running errands.
- Take a brisk walk during lunch breaks.
- Walk while taking phone calls or listening to podcasts.

3. Stand Instead of Sit

Why It Helps: Standing burns more calories than sitting and can improve posture and circulation.

How to Incorporate:

- Use a standing desk or alternate between sitting and standing while working.
- Stand while watching TV, folding laundry, or waiting in line.
- Make it a habit to stand up and stretch every 30 minutes.

4. Household Chores

Why It Helps: Cleaning, organizing, and doing laundry all require movement, which burns calories and keeps you active.

How to Incorporate:

- Tackle household tasks like vacuuming, mopping, or gardening.
- Set a timer for 10-15 minutes each day to tidy up your space.
- Turn cleaning into a mini workout by adding extra energy to your movements.

5. Stretching and Fidgeting

Why It Helps: Even small movements like stretching or fidgeting can increase your energy expenditure.

How to Incorporate:

- Stretch your arms, legs, and back during work breaks.
- Keep small exercise tools like resistance bands nearby for quick stretches.
- If you're seated, tap your feet, bounce your legs, or perform seated stretches.

6. Active Socializing

Why It Helps: Spending time with others in an active way, rather than sitting, can help burn more calories.

How to Incorporate:

- Invite friends for a walk instead of meeting for coffee.
- Play an active game like frisbee, badminton, or a casual sport.
- Take family outings to parks, zoos, or hiking trails.

7. Short Bursts of Exercise

Why It Helps: Incorporating short, 5-10 minute bursts of movement throughout the day can add up to a significant calorie burn.

How to Incorporate:

- Do a quick set of jumping jacks, squats, or push-ups during breaks.
- Incorporate a brief yoga or stretching routine in the morning or evening.
- Use commercials during TV shows as a cue to move.

How to Stay Consistent with Small Activities

1. **Set Reminders:**
   Use apps or alarms to remind yourself to stand, stretch, or walk throughout the day.
2. **Track Your Steps:**
   A fitness tracker or pedometer can help you monitor how much you're moving daily, motivating you to increase your activity.
3. **Pair Activities with Habits:**
   Combine small activities with daily habits, like squats while brushing your teeth or stretching while waiting for your coffee to brew.
4. **Make It Enjoyable:**
   Choose activities you find fun, such as dancing to your favorite songs or playing with pets.

The Cumulative Impact of Small Activities

Though these activities might seem minor, their cumulative impact can be significant. Over time, incorporating small movements throughout your day can increase your total daily energy expenditure, helping you burn more calories, improve your overall fitness, and maintain a healthy weight. These strategies not only support fat loss but also help combat the negative effects of prolonged sitting, contributing to better physical and mental health.

The Benefits of Walking, Biking, and Other Simple Movements

Incorporating simple, low-intensity movements like walking, biking, or even gardening into your daily routine can have profound health benefits. While these activities may not always feel like traditional exercise, they play a crucial role in maintaining overall health and contributing to calorie burn. Here's why these forms of movement are so effective and how they can fit into your lifestyle.

1. Accessible and Low-Impact Exercise

Walking and biking are among the most accessible forms of physical activity. They don't require specialized equipment (apart from a good pair of shoes or a bike) and can be done virtually anywhere. For people with joint pain or limited mobility, these low-impact exercises offer an excellent way to stay active without putting undue stress on the body. Activities like walking on soft surfaces or cycling on flat terrain are particularly gentle on the knees and hips.

2. Supports Cardiovascular Health

Even at a moderate pace, walking and biking help improve cardiovascular health by strengthening the heart, improving circulation, and lowering blood pressure. Regular cardiovascular exercise can also reduce the risk of chronic diseases such as heart disease, type 2 diabetes, and stroke. By engaging in simple movements consistently, you're giving your heart the workout it needs to stay strong.

3. Aids in Weight Management

While high-intensity exercises are known for burning a large number of calories in a short time, low-intensity activities like walking and biking can be just as effective over the long term.

Consistent movement throughout the day increases your non-exercise activity thermogenesis (NEAT), the energy expended for activities other than sleeping, eating, or sports-like exercise. Over time, these simple activities contribute significantly to calorie burn and help you maintain a healthy weight.

4. Boosts Mental Health and Mood

There's a strong link between physical activity and mental well-being, and walking or biking outdoors can provide an extra boost. Exposure to natural light and fresh air helps release endorphins, which improve mood and reduce stress and anxiety. Many people find that these activities provide a mental break from daily stressors, offering a meditative or calming experience.

5. Improves Muscular Endurance and Bone Health

Walking, especially on varied terrain, and biking help build and maintain muscular endurance, particularly in the lower body. These activities also contribute to bone health by stimulating bone density in weight-bearing areas such as the hips and legs. As a result, they reduce the risk of osteoporosis and other bone-related conditions.

6. Fits Seamlessly into Daily Life

One of the greatest advantages of simple movements is that they can easily fit into your daily routine. Walking to work, biking to the store, or taking a stroll during lunch breaks can significantly increase your daily activity level without requiring extra time. You can also combine these activities with social interactions, such as walking with friends or biking with family.

Practical Tips for Incorporating Simple Movements

- **Start Small**: Begin with a 10-15 minute walk or bike ride and gradually increase your time and distance.

- **Make It a Habit**: Incorporate walking or biking into your daily schedule by setting reminders or establishing a routine.
- **Track Your Progress**: Use a pedometer, fitness tracker, or app to monitor your steps or distance to stay motivated.
- **Explore New Routes**: Keep things interesting by changing your walking or biking paths regularly.

Setting Daily Movement Goals for Long-Term Success

In today's fast-paced world, finding time for physical activity can be challenging. However, staying active doesn't always mean spending hours in the gym. Incorporating daily movement goals into your routine is a practical and sustainable way to stay healthy, improve your fitness, and enhance your well-being over the long term. Here's how setting and sticking to daily movement goals can lead to lasting success.

1. The Importance of Daily Movement

Daily movement is essential for maintaining physical and mental health. Regular physical activity helps improve cardiovascular health, boost metabolism, enhance mood, and support weight management. Even small amounts of movement, when done consistently, can have significant long-term benefits. Setting daily goals encourages you to stay active and prevent the negative effects of a sedentary lifestyle, such as stiffness, reduced energy levels, and weight gain.

2. Start with Realistic Goals

When setting daily movement goals, it's important to start with realistic and achievable targets. Begin by assessing your current activity level and gradually increase your goals over time. For example, if you're currently sedentary, aim to take 5,000 steps a day, then gradually increase to 7,500 or 10,000 steps. The key is consistency rather than intensity, especially in the beginning.

3. Incorporate a Variety of Activities

Daily movement doesn't have to be monotonous. Incorporate a mix of activities to keep things interesting and engage different muscle groups. Walking, biking, stretching, or even short bodyweight exercises like squats or push-ups can all contribute to your movement goals. Variety helps prevent boredom and ensures that you're working different parts of your body, reducing the risk of overuse injuries.

4. Make It Part of Your Routine

One of the most effective ways to meet your daily movement goals is to make them part of your routine. Look for opportunities to add movement throughout your day. Take the stairs instead of the elevator, park farther away from entrances, or take short walking breaks during work hours. Establishing these habits makes daily activity feel natural rather than forced.

5. Use Technology to Stay Accountable

Technology can be a great ally in helping you stay on track. Fitness trackers and smartphone apps allow you to monitor your daily steps, active minutes, and calorie expenditure. Many devices also offer reminders to move if you've been inactive for too long. Seeing your progress in real-time can be motivating and help you stay accountable to your goals.

6. Celebrate Small Wins

Acknowledging and celebrating your progress is crucial for maintaining motivation. Each time you meet or exceed your daily movement goal, take a moment to celebrate. Small wins build confidence and create positive reinforcement, making it more likely that you'll stick with your routine in the long run.

7. Adapt Goals as Needed

Life can be unpredictable, and it's essential to adapt your goals as circumstances change. On busy or low-energy days, focus on lighter activities or shorter durations. Conversely, on days when you have more time or energy, you can aim for more intense or longer sessions. Flexibility ensures that you remain consistent without feeling overwhelmed.

Final Thoughts

Small activities throughout the day may not replace a dedicated workout, but they're an important supplement to an active lifestyle. By integrating simple movements like walking, standing, and doing chores, you can keep your metabolism active and enjoy the benefits of a more dynamic routine. Over time, these small changes can add up, making it easier to achieve and maintain your fitness goals without feeling overwhelmed. Remember, every bit of movement counts!

Simple movements like walking and biking may seem basic, but their benefits for physical and mental health are undeniable. These activities are accessible, sustainable, and highly effective for maintaining an active lifestyle. By embracing these low-impact forms of exercise, you can improve your cardiovascular health, boost your mood, and manage your weight without the need for an intense workout regime. Whether you're new to exercise or looking for easy ways to stay active, these simple movements can help you build a healthier, more balanced life.

Setting daily movement goals is a powerful strategy for achieving long-term health and fitness success. By starting small, incorporating variety, and celebrating your achievements, you can create a sustainable routine that keeps you active and engaged. Whether it's a short walk, a bike ride, or a few stretches, every bit of movement contributes to your overall well-being. Over time, these daily habits become a cornerstone of a healthier, more active lifestyle, helping you achieve your long-term health goals.

Part 3

Mindset, Motivation, and Sustainable Habits

Chapter 11

Setting Realistic Goals and Tracking Progress

Defining Your Why: The Key to Staying Motivated

Embarking on a health and fitness journey requires more than just a well-structured plan or a list of goals; it demands a strong sense of purpose. This is where defining your "why" comes into play. Your "why" is the deeply personal reason that fuels your drive, keeps you focused, and helps you overcome obstacles. It's the foundation of your motivation and the anchor that keeps you steady when challenges arise.

Why Your "Why" Matters

Many people start their fitness or weight loss journeys with external goals, such as fitting into a certain size or achieving a specific number on the scale. While these goals can be motivating in the short term, they often fail to sustain long-term commitment. When faced with setbacks or plateaus, it's easy to lose sight of why you started.

However, when you have a clear, emotionally resonant "why," you're more likely to stay committed. Whether your purpose is to improve your health for your family, feel more confident in your own skin, or enhance your quality of life, your "why" serves as a powerful motivator that transcends temporary struggles.

How to Discover Your Why

Finding your "why" involves introspection and self-awareness. Here's a step-by-step process to help you define it:

1. **Reflect on Your Values and Priorities:** Consider what matters most to you in life. Is it your family, your career,

or your long-term health? Think about how achieving your fitness goals aligns with these values. For example, improving your health may enable you to be more active with your kids or perform better at work.

2. **Ask Deep Questions:** Go beyond surface-level motivations. Instead of stopping at "I want to lose weight," ask yourself, *Why do I want to lose weight?* Perhaps it's to feel more energetic, to reduce the risk of chronic diseases, or to regain confidence. Keep digging until you reach a reason that resonates emotionally.

3. **Visualize Your Future Self:** Picture the version of yourself who has achieved these goals. What does your life look like? How do you feel physically and emotionally? This visualization can make your "why" more tangible and compelling.

4. **Write It Down:** Once you've defined your "why," write it down. This could be in the form of a statement or a few key points. Keep it somewhere visible, like on your fridge or in your workout space, to serve as a daily reminder.

Staying Connected to Your Why

Even with a clear "why," motivation can waver over time. Here's how to maintain a strong connection to your purpose:

1. **Revisit Your Why Regularly:** Set aside time to reflect on your "why" and how far you've come. This can help reignite your motivation during challenging times.

2. **Adapt as Needed:** Your goals and circumstances may change over time, and so might your "why." For instance, if you initially started your fitness journey to improve your appearance, you might later find that your motivation shifts toward enhancing your overall well-being or mental health.

3. **Celebrate Progress:** Recognize and celebrate milestones that align with your "why." This not only boosts your

confidence but also reinforces the importance of your journey.

4. **Seek Support:** Share your "why" with trusted friends, family members, or a fitness community. They can provide encouragement and remind you of your purpose when you need a boost.

How to Set SMART Goals for Weight Loss and Fitness

Setting clear and achievable goals is crucial for success in any fitness or weight loss journey. Without a defined target, it's easy to lose focus and motivation. That's where SMART goals come in. SMART stands for **Specific, Measurable, Achievable, Relevant, and Time-bound**. By adhering to this framework, you can create a roadmap for success that keeps you on track and motivated.

1. Specific: Define Clear, Concrete Goals

A specific goal provides a clear direction. Instead of saying, "I want to lose weight" or "I want to get fit," specify how much weight you want to lose or what fitness milestone you aim to achieve.

- **Example**: "I want to lose 10 pounds" or "I want to run a 5K without stopping."

2. Measurable: Track Your Progress

Measurable goals allow you to monitor your progress and adjust your plan if necessary. Use tools like a fitness tracker, a food diary, or even progress photos to quantify your achievements.

- **Example**: "I will lose 1-2 pounds per week" or "I will track my calorie intake daily."

3. Achievable: Set Realistic Goals Within Your Reach

While it's important to aim high, your goals should be realistic based on your current fitness level, lifestyle, and time constraints. Setting goals that are too ambitious can lead to frustration and burnout.

- **Example**: If you're new to fitness, start with a goal of exercising 3 times a week rather than every day.

4. Relevant: Align Goals with Your Personal Priorities

Your goals should align with what matters most to you. Whether your focus is improving health, increasing energy, or boosting confidence, setting goals relevant to your "why" ensures lasting motivation.

- **Example**: "I want to improve my stamina so I can play with my kids" or "I want to lower my cholesterol levels to improve my health."

5. Time-bound: Set a Deadline for Achievement

A time-bound goal creates a sense of urgency and helps you stay focused. Without a deadline, it's easy to procrastinate or lose track of progress.

- **Example**: "I will lose 10 pounds in 12 weeks" or "I will run a 5K in 3 months."

The Power of SMART Goals

By setting SMART goals, you transform vague aspirations into actionable plans. This method not only keeps you organized but also boosts your confidence as you check off milestones along the way. Regularly revisit and adjust your goals to stay aligned with your progress and changing needs, ensuring a sustainable and fulfilling fitness journey.

Progress Tracking: Using Measurements, Photos, and Journals

Tracking progress is a vital component of any weight loss or fitness journey. It not only helps you stay accountable but also provides tangible evidence of your improvements over time. By using a combination of measurements, photos, and journaling, you can monitor your progress from multiple angles, keeping motivation high and ensuring you're on the right path to achieving your goals.

1. Measurements: Quantifying Your Progress

Regularly taking physical measurements offers a clear and objective way to track changes in your body composition. This method goes beyond the scale, highlighting improvements in areas such as muscle gain or fat loss.

Key Areas to Measure:

- **Weight**: Weigh yourself weekly or bi-weekly to monitor trends.
- **Body Circumference**: Use a tape measure to track changes in specific areas:
    - Waist
    - Hips
    - Thighs
    - Arms
    - Chest
- **Body Fat Percentage**: If possible, use body fat calipers or a smart scale for a more detailed picture of fat loss.

Benefits of Measurements:

- Provides a comprehensive view of progress.
- Highlights improvements even when the scale doesn't change significantly.

- Helps in adjusting workout and diet plans for better results.

2. Photos: Visual Motivation

Progress photos are a powerful tool for visualizing changes that may not be evident in daily life. By comparing pictures over time, you can see subtle transformations that boost motivation and confidence.

How to Take Effective Progress Photos:

- **Consistency**: Take photos at regular intervals (e.g., every 2-4 weeks).
- **Lighting and Pose**: Use the same lighting, clothing, and poses to ensure consistency.
- **Angles**: Capture front, side, and back views to get a full picture of your progress.

Benefits of Photos:

- Provides a visual timeline of your journey.
- Highlights changes in posture, muscle tone, and overall physique.
- Serves as a motivating reminder of how far you've come.

3. Journals: Reflecting on Your Journey

A fitness or weight loss journal is an invaluable tool for tracking not only physical progress but also your mental and emotional journey. Journaling helps you stay organized, reflect on successes and challenges, and make informed adjustments.

What to Include in Your Journal:

- **Daily or Weekly Goals**: Document your SMART goals and track completion.

- **Exercise Logs**: Record workouts, including exercises, sets, reps, and duration.
- **Food Intake**: Keep a log of meals, snacks, and beverages to monitor nutritional habits.
- **Mood and Energy Levels**: Note how you feel each day to identify patterns and correlations with diet and exercise.
- **Achievements and Setbacks**: Celebrate wins and reflect on areas for improvement.

Benefits of Journals:

- Encourages mindfulness and accountability.
- Helps identify patterns and triggers affecting progress.
- Provides a record of strategies that work best for you.

Combining Tracking Methods for Maximum Results

Using measurements, photos, and journaling together provides a holistic approach to progress tracking. Each method offers unique insights that, when combined, give you a comprehensive understanding of your journey.

Example Tracking Routine:

- **Weekly**: Take weight and body measurements, write in your journal.
- **Bi-Weekly or Monthly**: Capture progress photos.
- **Daily**: Log meals, workouts, and mood in your journal.

Integrating The Smoothie Diet into Progress Tracking

Incorporating a tool like **The Smoothie Diet** can enhance your tracking journey. By documenting your smoothie intake in your journal, you can monitor how it affects your weight loss, energy levels, and overall health. This easy-to-make, nutrient-dense option can complement your exercise routine and help you stay consistent with your dietary goals.

Conclusion

Defining your "why" is a powerful step toward creating lasting change. It provides the emotional connection and purpose that can keep you motivated through highs and lows. When you pair a clear "why" with actionable strategies and supportive tools like The Smoothie Diet, you're setting yourself up for long-term success. Stay connected to your purpose, adapt as needed, and remember that every small step forward brings you closer to the healthier, happier version of yourself.

Tracking progress through measurements, photos, and journaling is an empowering way to stay motivated and ensure long-term success. These tools not only provide objective insights but also celebrate the smaller victories that lead to lasting change. By integrating these methods into your routine, you'll build a strong foundation for achieving your weight loss and fitness goals while maintaining a positive and motivated mindset.

Chapter 12

Overcoming Plateaus and Staying Motivated

Understanding Weight Loss Plateaus: What's Really Happening

Weight loss plateaus can be frustrating, but they are a normal and often misunderstood part of the journey. A plateau occurs when your weight loss stalls despite maintaining the same diet and exercise routine. Understanding the science behind plateaus can help you approach them with a balanced mindset and develop strategies to overcome them.

What Causes Weight Loss Plateaus?

1. **Metabolic Adaptation:** As you lose weight, your body requires fewer calories to function because it becomes more efficient. This is a survival mechanism designed to prevent excessive weight loss during times of scarcity. Your resting metabolic rate (RMR) decreases, meaning you burn fewer calories at rest. This can lead to a calorie balance where your intake matches your expenditure, halting weight loss.

2. **Loss of Water Weight and Glycogen:** In the initial stages of weight loss, a significant portion of the weight shed is water. As your body burns glycogen (stored carbohydrates) for energy, water is released. Over time, as your body depletes glycogen stores, further weight loss slows as fat becomes the primary source of energy.

3. **Muscle Gain or Retention:** If you've incorporated strength training into your routine, you might be gaining muscle mass. Since muscle is denser than fat, your weight might not change even though your body composition is improving. This can give the illusion of a plateau on the scale while your overall fitness is improving.

4. **Increased Caloric Intake:** Often, people unconsciously start eating more as they progress in their weight loss journey. This might be due to hunger cues triggered by increased activity levels or a psychological reward system for perceived progress. Even slight increases in calorie intake can offset your deficit and stall weight loss.

5. **Decreased Physical Activity:** As you lose weight, physical activities, including workouts and daily tasks, may burn fewer calories because of your lighter body. This reduction in calorie expenditure can also contribute to plateaus.

How to Overcome Weight Loss Plateaus

1. **Reassess Your Calorie Needs:** As your weight changes, your calorie needs adjust. Use an updated calorie calculator or consult a nutritionist to determine your new daily requirements. This might mean reducing your calorie intake slightly or increasing physical activity to maintain a deficit.

2. **Incorporate High-Intensity Workouts:** High-Intensity Interval Training (HIIT) or strength training can boost your metabolism and help overcome plateaus. These exercises promote muscle growth and increase the afterburn effect, where your body continues to burn calories post-workout.

3. **Mix Up Your Routine:** Your body adapts to repetitive exercise routines. Changing the intensity, duration, or type of workout can challenge your muscles and boost calorie burn. If you've been focusing on cardio, try adding strength training or vice versa.

4. **Focus on Non-Scale Victories:** Plateaus often occur on the scale, but other indicators like measurements, body fat percentage, or how your clothes fit may still show progress. Celebrate these victories to stay motivated.

5. **Practice Patience and Persistence:** Plateaus test your mental resilience. Remember that weight loss is not linear,

and temporary stalls are part of the process. Staying consistent with your healthy habits will eventually lead to progress.

The Role of The Smoothie Diet in Breaking Plateaus

Incorporating tools like *The Smoothie Diet* can help refresh your routine by introducing nutrient-dense, low-calorie meal options. These delicious, easy-to-make smoothies can help reduce calorie intake without sacrificing nutrition, giving your metabolism a gentle nudge to overcome a plateau.

Proven Strategies to Break Through Plateaus

Hitting a plateau during a weight loss or fitness journey is a common and often frustrating experience. However, plateaus are also a natural part of the process and an opportunity to evaluate and refine your approach. By understanding why plateaus happen and implementing effective strategies, you can jumpstart your progress and stay on track toward your goals. Here's a detailed guide on proven methods to break through plateaus.

1. Reassess Your Caloric Intake

As you lose weight, your body's energy needs decrease. This means that the calorie intake that initially helped you lose weight might now be enough to maintain your current weight. To continue losing, it may be necessary to recalculate your caloric needs and adjust your intake accordingly.

- **Track Your Food Intake**: Use a food diary or app to monitor your meals. This can help you spot any unintentional increases in calories, such as through extra snacking or portion sizes.
- **Adjust Caloric Deficit**: Calculate a new caloric deficit based on your current weight and goals. For most people, a 10-15% reduction in daily calories can help reignite weight loss without drastic changes.

2. Switch Up Your Exercise Routine

Over time, your body adapts to your workout routine, which can reduce its effectiveness. Mixing up your exercises challenges different muscles and increases calorie burn, making it easier to break through a plateau.

- **Incorporate HIIT (High-Intensity Interval Training)**: HIIT workouts involve short bursts of intense exercise followed by rest periods. This method increases heart rate, maximizes calorie burn, and boosts your metabolism for hours after you finish.

- **Focus on Strength Training**: Adding strength training to your routine helps build muscle, which increases your resting metabolic rate (RMR). The more muscle you have, the more calories you'll burn at rest, even when not exercising.
- **Try New Activities**: Consider trying a new activity like swimming, cycling, or kickboxing. New challenges engage different muscle groups and keep your workouts interesting and effective.

3. Increase Your Protein Intake

Protein is a key nutrient for weight loss and maintaining muscle mass, especially if you're engaging in strength training. It can also keep you feeling full longer, reducing overall calorie intake.

- **Include Protein in Every Meal**: Aim to include a source of lean protein in each meal and snack, such as chicken, fish, eggs, legumes, or tofu.
- **Use Protein to Curb Cravings**: Protein can help curb cravings for sweets or high-calorie snacks, which may help you stay on track with your goals.

4. Prioritize Sleep and Manage Stress

Poor sleep and high stress can significantly impact your body's ability to lose weight. Lack of sleep can lead to hormonal imbalances that affect hunger, and stress can trigger cravings for unhealthy foods.

- **Establish a Bedtime Routine**: Aim for 7-8 hours of sleep per night. Going to bed and waking up at the same time each day can help regulate your sleep cycle.
- **Incorporate Stress-Reduction Techniques**: Try mindfulness practices, yoga, or breathing exercises to reduce stress levels. Regular stress management helps

maintain balanced cortisol levels, which can support weight loss.

5. Focus on Non-Scale Victories

Plateaus often happen on the scale, but other forms of progress may still be occurring. Celebrating these wins can help keep you motivated and engaged in your journey.

- **Take Measurements and Photos**: Muscle gain or fat loss may not show on the scale but will be evident in body measurements and photos. Track progress in inches lost, improved muscle tone, or how clothes fit.
- **Track Fitness Progress**: Monitor increases in strength, endurance, or flexibility. Improvements in fitness levels indicate progress even if the scale doesn't budge.

6. Use The Smoothie Diet as a Refreshing Reset

Including a program like *The Smoothie Diet* can help you break through a plateau by providing nutrient-dense, low-calorie meal options. These smoothies are quick to make and can help you stay satisfied while reducing your overall calorie intake. Plus, they're packed with fiber, protein, and vitamins to support metabolism and energy levels, making it easier to stay on track with your goals.

7. Increase Daily Activity and NEAT

NEAT, or non-exercise activity thermogenesis, is the energy expended for daily tasks that aren't formal exercise, like walking, cleaning, or standing. Increasing NEAT can help boost calorie burn throughout the day.

- **Take the Stairs**: Opt for stairs instead of the elevator to add some extra movement.
- **Walk More Often**: Take short breaks to walk, especially if you have a sedentary job.

- **Stand Instead of Sitting**: Standing burns more calories than sitting and can help maintain energy levels throughout the day.

8. Stay Patient and Trust the Process

Breaking through a plateau requires persistence and a positive mindset. Remember, progress may not always be linear, and minor setbacks are natural. Maintaining a balanced approach and being patient with yourself can prevent burnout and keep you motivated over the long term.

How to Keep Motivation High When Progress Slows

Slowing progress, whether in weight loss or fitness, can be discouraging. However, it's important to recognize that periods of slower progress are normal and can even serve as opportunities for growth. Maintaining motivation during these times is crucial for long-term success. Here are practical strategies to help you stay focused and committed when your progress seems to stall.

1. Revisit Your "Why"

Your initial motivation likely stemmed from a specific reason or goal—whether it was improving your health, boosting your energy, or fitting into a favorite outfit. When progress slows, revisiting your "why" can help reignite your passion and commitment.

- **Write It Down**: Keep a journal of why you started your journey and revisit it frequently.
- **Visual Reminders**: Place motivating quotes, photos, or notes in places you see daily, like your fridge or bathroom mirror.

2. Set New, Short-Term Goals

Long-term goals are essential, but short-term goals can provide the immediate gratification needed to keep motivation high.

- **Break Down Big Goals**: Instead of focusing solely on losing 20 pounds, aim to lose 1-2 pounds per week.
- **Fitness Milestones**: If weight loss has slowed, focus on performance goals, like running a faster mile, lifting heavier weights, or completing more push-ups.

3. Celebrate Non-Scale Victories (NSVs)

Progress isn't always reflected on the scale. Non-scale victories can provide a sense of accomplishment and keep you motivated.

- **Improved Fitness**: Notice improvements in your endurance, strength, or flexibility.
- **Better Sleep and Energy Levels**: Acknowledge increased energy or better sleep quality as a result of your healthier habits.
- **Clothing Fit**: Pay attention to how your clothes fit, which may indicate body composition changes even if your weight remains the same.

4. Change Up Your Routine

Monotony can lead to boredom, making it harder to stay motivated. A fresh routine can reinvigorate your journey and push past slow progress.

- **Try New Workouts**: Swap your usual treadmill session for a dance class, swimming, or cycling.
- **Modify Intensity**: Incorporate high-intensity interval training (HIIT) or increase the resistance and weight in strength training.
- **Explore New Recipes**: Introduce variety in your diet with new, healthy recipes, like incorporating *The Smoothie Diet* for delicious, nutrient-packed meal options.

5. Find a Support System

Connecting with others who share similar goals can provide encouragement and accountability.

- **Workout Buddy**: Exercising with a friend can make workouts more enjoyable and help you stay consistent.

- **Online Communities**: Join fitness or health-related groups on social media for motivation and tips from people on similar journeys.
- **Hire a Coach or Trainer**: A professional can help adjust your program and keep you motivated when progress slows.

6. Focus on Building Habits, Not Just Outcomes

Consistent habits are the foundation of lasting success. Shifting your focus from outcomes to behaviors can reduce frustration and keep motivation high.

- **Daily Habits**: Commit to small, daily actions like drinking enough water, eating a balanced diet, and moving your body.
- **Reward Consistency**: Celebrate sticking to your plan, even if the results aren't immediately visible.

7. Practice Gratitude and Positive Self-Talk

Focusing on what your body can do rather than what it hasn't achieved can shift your perspective and maintain motivation.

- **Gratitude Journal**: Write down three things you're grateful for each day, focusing on your health and progress.
- **Positive Affirmations**: Replace negative self-talk with affirmations like, "I am strong," "I am making progress," or "I'm proud of my effort."

8. Be Patient and Trust the Process

Progress often comes in waves. Staying patient and committed, even during slower periods, ensures long-term success.

- **Understand Plateaus**: Recognize that plateaus are a normal part of any fitness or weight loss journey.
- **Focus on the Big Picture**: Remember that health and fitness are lifelong pursuits, not short-term fixes.

Conclusion

Weight loss plateaus are a natural part of the journey and an opportunity to reassess and refine your approach. By understanding the science behind them and applying practical strategies, you can navigate plateaus with confidence and continue your progress toward your weight loss goals.

Plateaus are a normal part of the weight loss journey but don't have to be a roadblock. By recalculating your calorie intake, adjusting your workout routine, managing stress, focusing on non-scale victories, and possibly incorporating The Smoothie Diet for a nutritious reset, you can overcome plateaus and continue progressing toward your goals. With consistency, adaptability, and a positive approach, you'll be well-equipped to keep seeing results on your journey.

Keeping motivation high when progress slows requires a blend of mindset shifts, habit reinforcement, and strategic adjustments. By revisiting your goals, celebrating non-scale victories, staying consistent with your habits, and seeking support, you can overcome the mental hurdles of slower progress. Remember, every small step counts, and with perseverance, your long-term health and fitness goals remain within reach.

Chapter 13

Creating Lasting Healthy Habits

The Science of Habit Formation and How to Make Changes Stick

Creating lasting healthy habits is a fundamental aspect of achieving long-term wellness. However, building these habits requires understanding the science of habit formation and applying strategies that help new behaviors stick. By learning how habits work and how to structure your environment and mindset, you can make meaningful, sustainable changes to your lifestyle.

Understanding the Habit Loop: Cue, Routine, Reward

At the core of habit formation lies the **habit loop**, a cycle consisting of three components:

1. **Cue:** A trigger that initiates the behavior. It could be time of day, location, emotional state, or a specific event.
   - Example: Seeing your running shoes by the door reminds you to go for a jog.
2. **Routine:** The actual behavior or action.
   - Example: Jogging for 30 minutes.
3. **Reward:** The positive outcome that reinforces the habit.
   - Example: Feeling energized and accomplished after the run.

By understanding this loop, you can intentionally design habits by identifying specific cues and rewards to reinforce your desired routines.

The Role of Repetition and Consistency

Habits are formed through **repetition**. Research shows that repeating a behavior in the same context helps solidify the connection between the cue and the routine. On average, it takes **21 to 66 days** to form a new habit, depending on the complexity of the behavior and individual differences.

Tips for Building Consistency:

- Start small: Focus on simple, manageable habits that are easy to incorporate into your daily routine.
- Stack habits: Attach a new habit to an existing one. For example, do a short meditation after brushing your teeth.
- Set reminders: Use alarms, sticky notes, or habit-tracking apps to stay on track.

The Importance of Motivation and Identity

Motivation plays a critical role in initiating new habits, but long-term success often requires tying the habit to your **identity**. Instead of focusing solely on outcomes, align your habits with the type of person you want to become.

Shift Your Mindset:

- **Outcome-based approach**: "I want to lose 10 pounds."
- **Identity-based approach**: "I am someone who prioritizes health and fitness."

This identity-based framework helps internalize the habit, making it part of your self-concept and reducing the reliance on external motivation.

Overcoming Challenges and Staying Flexible

Forming new habits isn't always smooth. Obstacles such as lack of time, stress, or competing priorities can derail progress.

Anticipating these challenges and developing strategies to navigate them is crucial.

Strategies to Overcome Barriers:

- **Plan for setbacks**: Expect that life will disrupt your routine occasionally. Instead of feeling discouraged, focus on getting back on track quickly.
- **Adjust as needed**: If a habit isn't working, tweak it. For example, if morning workouts are difficult, try exercising in the evening.
- **Reward progress**: Celebrate small wins to maintain motivation.

Making Changes Stick: Long-Term Strategies

1. **Environment Design**: Shape your surroundings to support your habits.
   o Example: Keep healthy snacks visible and junk food out of sight.
2. **Social Support**: Surround yourself with people who share your goals or encourage your progress.
   o Join fitness classes, online communities, or workout with a friend.
3. **Reflection and Tracking**: Regularly review your progress using journals, apps, or other tracking tools.
   o Track metrics like workout frequency, water intake, or hours of sleep.
4. **Revisit Your Why**: Periodically remind yourself why you started. Reflecting on your motivations helps sustain commitment.

Tips for Building and Maintaining a Healthy Routine

Building and maintaining a healthy routine is essential for long-term well-being. Whether your goal is to improve your physical fitness, enhance mental health, or achieve better work-life balance, a structured routine helps create consistency and stability in your daily life. This guide offers practical tips for establishing and sustaining habits that support a healthier, more fulfilling lifestyle.

1. Start with Small, Achievable Goals

One of the biggest mistakes when creating a healthy routine is trying to change everything at once. Instead, focus on small, incremental changes that are easy to implement and maintain.

- **Break Down Larger Goals**: If your goal is to exercise regularly, start with 10-minute sessions a few times a week and gradually increase the duration and frequency.
- **Celebrate Small Wins**: Each milestone you achieve reinforces your commitment and builds momentum.

2. Create a Structured Daily Plan

A clear daily schedule helps ensure that healthy habits become part of your routine. Allocate specific times for key activities, such as exercise, meal prep, and relaxation.

- **Use Tools**: Utilize calendars, planners, or habit-tracking apps to organize your day.
- **Prioritize Key Activities**: Identify non-negotiable habits, such as getting enough sleep or staying hydrated, and make them a priority.

3. Incorporate Variety

A monotonous routine can lead to burnout or boredom, which might cause you to abandon healthy habits. Including variety keeps your routine fresh and engaging.

- **Mix Up Your Workouts**: Alternate between cardio, strength training, and flexibility exercises.
- **Try New Recipes**: Experiment with different healthy meals to keep your diet interesting and enjoyable.

4. Set Reminders and Triggers

Habits thrive on consistency, and setting reminders can help reinforce new behaviors until they become second nature.

- **Use Visual Cues**: Place workout gear where you can see it or keep a water bottle on your desk as a reminder to hydrate.
- **Schedule Notifications**: Set alarms or reminders on your phone for key activities, like stretching breaks or bedtime.

5. Stay Flexible and Adapt

Life is unpredictable, and rigid routines can be challenging to maintain when circumstances change. Flexibility is crucial for long-term success.

- **Adapt to Your Needs**: If you're feeling fatigued, swap a high-intensity workout for a lighter activity like yoga or a walk.
- **Adjust for Life Events**: Modify your routine during busy periods, such as holidays or work deadlines, but aim to maintain the core elements.

6. Seek Accountability and Support

Having a support system can significantly enhance your ability to stick to a healthy routine. Sharing your goals with others provides motivation and accountability.

- **Buddy Up**: Partner with a friend or family member to exercise or cook healthy meals together.
- **Join a Community**: Participate in fitness classes, wellness groups, or online forums for additional encouragement and support.

7. Prioritize Rest and Recovery

Rest is as important as activity in any healthy routine. Overworking your body or mind can lead to burnout, diminishing the effectiveness of your efforts.

- **Get Adequate Sleep**: Aim for 7-9 hours of quality sleep each night to support physical and mental recovery.
- **Schedule Downtime**: Incorporate relaxation techniques like meditation, deep breathing, or leisurely walks into your routine.

8. Evaluate and Adjust Regularly

A healthy routine should evolve over time to meet your changing needs and goals. Regularly assessing your progress helps ensure you're on the right track.

- **Reflect Weekly**: Take time each week to review what's working and what's not.
- **Set New Challenges**: Once a habit feels ingrained, challenge yourself with new goals, such as increasing workout intensity or trying a different form of exercise.

9. Make it Enjoyable

For a routine to be sustainable, it should bring joy and satisfaction. If you dread a particular activity, you're less likely to stick with it.

- **Find Activities You Love**: Choose exercises, hobbies, or meal options that you genuinely enjoy.
- **Reward Yourself**: Treat yourself to non-food rewards, like new workout gear or a relaxing massage, for staying consistent.

How to Enjoy the Process and Celebrate Your Wins

Creating lasting healthy habits is not just about discipline and consistency; it's also about finding joy in the journey and celebrating milestones along the way. Enjoying the process helps you stay motivated and reinforces positive behavior, making it easier to sustain your efforts over the long term. Here's how to embrace the journey and acknowledge your successes.

1. Shift Your Mindset: Focus on Growth, Not Perfection

Adopting a growth mindset means viewing challenges and setbacks as opportunities to learn rather than as failures.

- **Embrace Progress Over Perfection**: Understand that small improvements, like choosing a healthier snack or taking the stairs, are victories.
- **Celebrate Effort, Not Just Results**: Recognize the hard work and dedication you're putting into building healthier habits, regardless of immediate outcomes.

2. Find Activities You Enjoy

Healthy habits are more sustainable when they're enjoyable. Incorporating activities that you look forward to can transform your routine from a chore into a source of joy.

- **Experiment with Different Workouts**: Try yoga, dance, swimming, or hiking until you find something you love.
- **Make Meal Prep Fun**: Explore new recipes, involve friends or family, or listen to your favorite music or podcast while cooking.

3. Set Mini-Milestones and Celebrate Small Wins

Breaking larger goals into smaller milestones makes them more manageable and provides regular opportunities to celebrate.

- **Acknowledge Daily Wins**: Whether it's drinking more water, completing a workout, or sticking to your meal plan, recognize these achievements.
- **Reward Yourself**: Treat yourself to non-food rewards like a relaxing bath, a new book, or workout gear to mark your progress.

4. Track and Reflect on Your Progress

Keeping track of your journey helps you see how far you've come and keeps you motivated to continue.

- **Use a Journal or App**: Record your workouts, meals, and mood changes to visualize your progress.
- **Reflect on Achievements**: At the end of each week or month, take time to look back at what you've accomplished.

5. Celebrate Non-Scale Victories (NSVs)

Weight loss and fitness goals often focus on numbers, but non-scale victories are equally important.

- **Improved Energy Levels**: Feeling more energetic throughout the day.
- **Enhanced Mood and Mental Clarity**: Noticing reduced stress or increased focus.
- **Physical Milestones**: Completing a longer run, lifting heavier weights, or mastering a yoga pose.

6. Practice Gratitude

Gratitude can shift your focus from what you haven't achieved to what you have. It helps you appreciate the journey and stay positive.

- **Daily Gratitude Practice**: Write down three things you're grateful for each day, related to your health journey.
- **Celebrate Your Body**: Appreciate what your body can do, rather than solely focusing on appearance.

7. Build a Support Network

Surrounding yourself with supportive people can make the journey more enjoyable and help you stay accountable.

- **Share Your Wins**: Celebrate successes with friends, family, or a fitness community.
- **Encourage Others**: Helping someone else achieve their goals can also be rewarding and motivating for you.

8. Keep It Fun and Creative

Staying engaged and excited about your routine is key to enjoying the process.

- **Ga mify Your Goals**: Set up challenges for yourself, like hitting a certain number of steps or trying a new workout each week.
- **Mix Things Up**: Avoid monotony by varying your exercises, trying new healthy recipes, or exploring different forms of relaxation like meditation or journaling.

9. Celebrate Your Journey, Not Just the Destination

Remember that the path to better health is ongoing. Celebrate not only reaching your goals but also the lifestyle changes and mindset shifts you've adopted along the way.

- **Host a Celebration**: When you hit a major milestone, celebrate with loved ones or treat yourself to a special experience.

- **Recognize Your Resilience**: Take pride in the fact that you're committing to your well-being, even on tough days.

Conclusion

Understanding the science of habit formation empowers you to take control of your behaviors and create lasting, positive changes. By leveraging the habit loop, building consistency, aligning habits with your identity, and staying adaptable, you can develop routines that enhance your well-being. Remember, lasting habits are not formed overnight but through persistent effort and mindful adjustments.

Building and maintaining a healthy routine requires intention, effort, and flexibility. By starting small, structuring your day, and finding joy in the process, you can create sustainable habits that support your overall health and well-being. Remember, progress takes time, and every step you take toward consistency contributes to long-term success.

Enjoying the process and celebrating your wins is essential to creating lasting healthy habits. By focusing on what you love, acknowledging progress, and rewarding yourself, you'll make your health journey not just sustainable but deeply fulfilling. Remember, every step forward is a reason to celebrate, and the joy you find in the journey will carry you toward long-term success.

Part 4
Putting It All Together

Chapter 14

Your 30-Day Fit & Fueled Plan

A Step-by-Step Plan for Getting Started

Embarking on a 30-day journey toward better fitness and nutrition can be transformative, but it requires a clear plan to set yourself up for success. Whether you're looking to lose weight, build muscle, or improve your overall health, a structured approach ensures that your goals are achievable and sustainable. Here's a comprehensive step-by-step plan to help you get started on your 30-day Fit & Fueled Plan.

1. Define Your Goals and Motivation

Before beginning any fitness or nutrition plan, it's essential to understand why you're doing it.

- **Set Clear Goals**: Identify what you want to achieve in the next 30 days. Examples include losing a certain amount of weight, increasing strength, or improving endurance.
- **Define Your 'Why'**: Reflect on why these goals matter to you—whether it's improving your health, boosting your confidence, or setting a positive example for loved ones.

2. Assess Your Current Fitness and Nutrition Levels

Understanding your starting point helps tailor your plan.

- **Track Your Current Habits**: Spend a few days observing your eating patterns, physical activity, and sleep schedule.

- **Take Baseline Measurements**: Record your weight, body measurements, and fitness benchmarks (like how many push-ups or minutes of cardio you can do).

3. Plan Your Workouts

- Designing a balanced exercise routine is crucial for success. Aim to include cardio, strength training, and flexibility exercises.

- **Week 1-2**: Start with moderate-intensity workouts 3-4 times a week. Incorporate both cardio (e.g., brisk walking, cycling) and basic strength training exercises (e.g., bodyweight squats, push-ups).
- **Week 3-4**: Gradually increase workout intensity and frequency. Add variety to keep things exciting, such as interval training or trying new workout styles like yoga or pilates.
- **Rest Days**: Schedule at least one rest or active recovery day per week to allow your body to recover and prevent burnout.

4. Create a Nutrition Plan

Fueling your body with the right foods is just as important as exercise.

- **Focus on Whole Foods**: Prioritize lean proteins, whole grains, fruits, vegetables, and healthy fats.
- **Meal Prep**: Dedicate time each week to plan and prepare meals. This ensures you always have healthy options available.
- **Incorporate The Smoothie Diet**: A simple, tasty way to boost your nutrition is by replacing one meal a day with a nutrient-packed smoothie. This can help with weight loss while ensuring you get essential vitamins and minerals.

5. Set Daily and Weekly Milestones

Breaking your 30-day plan into smaller milestones helps you stay on track and celebrate progress.

- **Daily Goals**: Include actions like drinking 8 glasses of water, completing a workout, or preparing a healthy meal.
- **Weekly Goals**: Track bigger milestones, such as completing all scheduled workouts or sticking to your meal plan.

6. Track Your Progress

Regularly monitoring your efforts keeps you motivated and helps identify areas for improvement.

- **Use a Journal or App**: Record your workouts, meals, and how you feel each day.
- **Take Progress Photos**: Visual changes often provide motivation that the scale doesn't capture.
- **Review Weekly**: Set aside time to reflect on your achievements and adjust your plan as needed.

7. Stay Accountable

Accountability can significantly increase your chances of success.

- **Find a Workout Buddy**: Exercising with a friend makes it more enjoyable and helps you stay committed.
- **Join Online Communities**: Connect with others following similar plans for motivation and support.
- **Check-In Regularly**: Share your progress with a coach, friend, or family member.

8. Overcome Challenges

Anticipate and plan for potential obstacles.

- **Identify Triggers**: Recognize situations that lead to unhealthy choices and create strategies to manage them.
- **Plan for Busy Days**: Have quick, healthy meals and shorter workout options ready for when time is limited.
- **Practice Mindset Shifts**: View setbacks as opportunities to learn and grow rather than failures.

9. Celebrate Your Wins

Acknowledging progress, no matter how small, keeps motivation high.

- **Reward Yourself**: Treat yourself to non-food rewards like new workout gear, a massage, or a fun outing.
- **Celebrate Milestones**: Reaching a weight goal, increasing strength, or simply sticking to the plan for 30 days are all reasons to celebrate.

10. Plan for Post-30 Days

The end of your 30-day plan doesn't mean the end of your journey.

- **Reflect on Your Experience**: Identify what worked well and what could be improved.
- **Set New Goals**: Build on your progress by setting new, achievable targets for the next phase.
- **Maintain Healthy Habits**: Incorporate what you've learned into your daily routine for long-term success.

Nutrition and Exercise Plans for Different Fitness Levels

Every individual embarks on their fitness journey from a unique starting point, with varying levels of experience, stamina, and goals. Whether you're a beginner, intermediate, or advanced athlete, tailoring your nutrition and exercise plan to your current fitness level is essential for sustainable progress. Incorporating a well-balanced diet, such as The Smoothie Diet, can complement your efforts, providing essential nutrients to fuel your workouts and support recovery.

1. For Beginners

Exercise Plan:
Starting out, the focus should be on building a solid foundation with low-impact exercises that promote consistency and prevent injury.

- **Cardio:** Aim for 20-30 minutes of moderate cardio, such as brisk walking, cycling, or swimming, 3-4 times a week.
- **Strength Training:** Begin with bodyweight exercises (e.g., squats, lunges, push-ups) twice a week.
- **Flexibility:** Incorporate stretching or yoga 2-3 times a week to improve mobility and reduce stiffness.

Nutrition Plan:
For beginners, the goal is to develop healthy eating habits. This is where The Smoothie Diet can be a game-changer. By replacing one or two meals a day with nutrient-packed smoothies, you can easily control calorie intake while ensuring your body gets essential vitamins and minerals. Pair this with whole grains, lean proteins, and plenty of vegetables.

2. For Intermediate Level

Exercise Plan:
Intermediate individuals can handle a more structured workout routine with increased intensity.

- **Cardio:** Include 30-45 minutes of varied cardio (e.g., jogging, interval training) 4-5 times a week.
- **Strength Training:** Focus on resistance training 3-4 times weekly, incorporating both bodyweight and free weights to challenge muscles.
- **Flexibility & Recovery:** Stretching, foam rolling, or yoga at least 3 times a week to aid in recovery and flexibility.

Nutrition Plan:
At this level, macronutrient balance becomes more critical. Along with using The Smoothie Diet for convenient, energy-boosting meals, focus on portion control. Increase protein intake to support muscle recovery, and include healthy fats for sustained energy. Meal prepping can help ensure you stick to your nutrition plan during busy weeks.

3. For Advanced Level

Exercise Plan:
Advanced fitness enthusiasts often aim for peak performance and specific goals such as muscle gain or endurance.

- **Cardio:** Incorporate high-intensity interval training (HIIT) or long-distance running 5-6 times a week.
- **Strength Training:** Engage in advanced weightlifting techniques (e.g., supersets, heavy lifting) 4-5 times a week.
- **Flexibility & Mobility:** Include dynamic stretching, advanced yoga, or Pilates sessions to maintain flexibility and prevent injuries.

Nutrition Plan:
Precision and timing are crucial at this level. The Smoothie Diet can serve as a perfect pre- or post-workout meal, providing quick and easily digestible nutrients to fuel intense training. Advanced athletes should focus on fine-tuning their macronutrient ratios based on their goals, whether it's fat loss, muscle gain, or improved endurance.

Weekly Check-ins and Adjustments: Staying on Track for Success

Embarking on a 30-day fitness and nutrition plan requires commitment, but it's equally important to remain flexible and adaptable. Weekly check-ins allow you to assess your progress, make necessary adjustments, and stay aligned with your goals. These regular evaluations ensure that your plan remains effective and tailored to your evolving needs, helping you maintain momentum and avoid plateaus.

Why Weekly Check-ins Matter

1. **Track Progress:** Weekly reviews give you the chance to monitor your weight, energy levels, workout performance, and overall well-being. By keeping tabs on these metrics, you can identify patterns and determine what's working or where adjustments are needed.
2. **Stay Accountable:** Setting aside time each week to reflect on your actions reinforces accountability. It's a structured moment to evaluate your adherence to the plan and re-commit to your goals.
3. **Identify Challenges Early:** Weekly check-ins help pinpoint obstacles before they become major setbacks. Whether it's a busy schedule, fatigue, or waning motivation, identifying issues early allows for proactive solutions.

Key Areas to Evaluate During Check-ins

1. **Nutrition:** Reflect on your meal choices over the past week. Have you been meeting your nutritional needs? If cravings or unhealthy habits have crept in, consider integrating The Smoothie Diet. These easy-to-make, nutrient-packed smoothies can help you stay on track by satisfying your hunger while supporting weight loss and energy levels.

2. **Exercise Performance:** Assess your workout routine. Are you hitting your fitness goals, whether it's increasing strength, endurance, or flexibility? If certain exercises feel too easy or too challenging, adjust your plan to better suit your fitness level.
3. **Mindset and Motivation:** Check in with your mental health and motivation. Are you feeling positive about your progress, or have you hit a motivational slump? Use this time to revisit your "why" and celebrate small wins to reignite your drive.
4. **Physical Changes and Energy Levels:** Notice how your body feels. Are you more energized or experiencing fatigue? Are you seeing changes in your physique, such as increased muscle tone or weight loss? These observations can guide your next steps.

Making Adjustments for Continued Progress

1. **Modify Nutrition Goals:** If weight loss has stalled or you're not feeling energized, tweak your calorie intake or nutrient balance. Including The Smoothie Diet in your plan can be a convenient adjustment to boost your nutrient intake and help you stay full longer without compromising your goals.
2. **Revise Workout Intensity:** Based on your performance, you may need to increase or decrease the intensity of your workouts. If cardio sessions feel too easy, increase duration or intensity. If strength training isn't challenging enough, try heavier weights or new exercises.
3. **Adapt to Life's Demands:** Life happens—travel, work deadlines, or family responsibilities can disrupt your routine. Use check-ins to recalibrate. Shorter workouts, meal prep, or focusing on active recovery can keep you moving forward.

Final Thoughts

A successful 30-day Fit & Fueled Plan combines clear goals, a structured workout and nutrition plan, and consistent progress tracking. By staying motivated, overcoming challenges, and celebrating your wins, you'll set a strong foundation for lasting health and fitness. With a positive mindset and the right strategies in place, this 30-day journey can be the start of a lifelong commitment to well-being.

No matter your fitness level, the combination of tailored exercise and nutrition plans is the key to achieving your goals. Weekly check-ins and adjustments are your roadmap to long-term success. By consistently evaluating your progress and making thoughtful changes, you can stay motivated and achieve your fitness goals.

Chapter 15

Long-Term Success and Maintenance

How to Transition from Weight Loss to Maintenance Mode

Understanding the Transition Phase

1. **Adjusting Caloric Intake**
   During weight loss, you likely consumed fewer calories to create a deficit. In maintenance mode, the goal is to find your *maintenance calorie level*—the number of calories your body needs to sustain your current weight without gaining or losing. Gradually increase your calorie intake by 100-200 calories per week until you notice your weight stabilizing.

2. **Prioritizing Nutrient-Dense Foods**
   Even as you increase calories, focus on nutrient-dense options that provide vitamins, minerals, and fiber. This helps maintain energy levels, supports overall health, and keeps you feeling full and satisfied.

3. **Maintaining an Active Lifestyle**
   Continue to include both cardio and strength training in your routine. Exercise helps regulate your metabolism and prevents weight regain by preserving lean muscle mass and promoting fat burning.

The Role of The Smoothie Diet in Maintenance Mode

The Smoothie Diet, which offers a variety of nutrient-dense and easy-to-make options, is a great tool for maintaining long-term success. It allows you to enjoy delicious meals while controlling portions and meeting your nutritional needs. Incorporate these smoothies as part of your daily meals or snacks to ensure you stay on track:

- **Breakfast Smoothies:** Kickstart your day with energy-boosting, high-fiber options.
- **Post-Workout Smoothies:** Replenish nutrients and support muscle recovery.
- **Meal Replacement Smoothies:** Provide balanced nutrition on busy days to prevent overeating.

By keeping smoothies as a staple in your diet, you'll have a convenient, healthy option that supports weight maintenance without compromising on taste.

Strategies for Long-Term Success in Maintenance Mode

1. **Monitor Your Weight and Adjust Accordingly**
   Regularly weigh yourself or use other progress indicators like how your clothes fit. Small fluctuations are normal, but significant changes may require adjustments to your calorie intake or exercise routine.

2. **Stay Mindful of Portions**
   Maintenance doesn't mean returning to old eating habits. Continue to practice portion control and mindful eating to prevent unconscious overeating.

3. **Focus on Sustainable Habits**
   The habits that helped you lose weight—like meal prepping, regular exercise, and hydration—are just as

important in maintenance mode. These practices form the foundation of a healthy lifestyle.

4. **Set New Goals Beyond Weight**
   To stay motivated, shift your focus from weight loss to other health-related goals, such as improving strength, increasing flexibility, or enhancing endurance. This keeps you engaged and excited about your fitness journey.

5. **Indulge Smartly**
   Allow yourself occasional treats while maintaining overall balance. The key is moderation, ensuring that indulgences don't derail your progress.

The Psychological Shift: Embracing Maintenance

Transitioning to maintenance requires a change in mindset. Instead of aiming for weight loss, the goal becomes sustaining your achievements. This shift can be empowering, as it emphasizes the importance of balance, enjoyment, and long-term health.

- **Celebrate Your Journey:** Reflect on how far you've come and acknowledge your hard work.
- **Find Joy in Routine:** Embrace the habits that make you feel good and fit seamlessly into your lifestyle.
- **Stay Connected to Your "Why":** Remember the reasons you started this journey, whether for health, confidence, or overall well-being.

Dealing with Setbacks and Staying Consistent

Setbacks are a natural part of any long-term journey, including maintaining weight loss and a healthy lifestyle. Whether it's a holiday indulgence, a busy period at work, or a temporary lapse in motivation, setbacks don't have to derail your progress. Instead, they can become opportunities to learn, grow, and strengthen your commitment to long-term success. By adopting a flexible mindset and practical strategies, you can navigate setbacks while staying consistent.

Understanding Setbacks: Why They Happen

1. **Life Circumstances**
   Changes in routine, such as vacations, social events, or personal challenges, can disrupt your healthy habits.
2. **Emotional Triggers**
   Stress, boredom, or emotional distress can lead to overeating or skipping workouts as coping mechanisms.
3. **Plateaus or Slower Progress**
   When progress slows, it's easy to feel discouraged, leading to a loss of motivation or reverting to old habits.
4. **Over-Reliance on Perfection**
   Striving for perfection often sets unrealistic expectations. A single slip-up can feel like failure, leading to more setbacks.

Strategies for Overcoming Setbacks

1. **Reframe Your Mindset**
   View setbacks as part of the process, not as failures. They are temporary and can provide valuable insights into what works for you and what doesn't.
2. **Identify Triggers**
   Reflect on what caused the setback. Was it a specific situation, emotion, or change in routine? Understanding the root cause helps you develop strategies to address similar challenges in the future.

3. **Practice Self-Compassion**

   Avoid harsh self-criticism. Treat yourself with the same kindness and encouragement you would offer a friend. Recognize that everyone faces setbacks.

4. **Set Small, Achievable Goals**

   Break your goals into manageable steps to regain momentum. For example, instead of aiming to return to a full workout routine immediately, commit to a 10-minute walk or one healthy meal per day.

Building Resilience and Consistency

1. **Create a Support System**

   Surround yourself with supportive friends, family, or a fitness community. Sharing your journey and challenges can help you stay accountable and motivated.

2. **Focus on Habits, Not Outcomes**

   Instead of fixating on the scale or immediate results, concentrate on the habits that lead to long-term success, such as regular exercise, balanced meals, and hydration.

3. **Celebrate Small Wins**

   Acknowledge and celebrate small achievements, even if they seem minor. Progress isn't always linear, and every step forward counts.

4. **Develop a Flexible Routine**

   Life is unpredictable, so having a flexible routine ensures you can adapt without losing consistency. For example, have a set of go-to home workouts or quick, healthy meal options like smoothies for days when time is limited.

5. **Plan for Setbacks**

   Anticipate situations where setbacks are likely, such as holidays or busy workweeks. Have a plan in place, like preparing healthy snacks or scheduling shorter workouts, to minimize their impact.

Maintaining Motivation Over the Long Term

1. **Reconnect with Your "Why"**
   Regularly remind yourself of the reasons you embarked on this journey, whether for improved health, increased confidence, or more energy for daily activities.
2. **Visualize Your Success**
   Imagine how you'll feel and what you'll achieve by staying consistent. Visualization can reinforce your commitment and inspire you to keep going.
3. **Embrace the Journey**
   Health and fitness are lifelong pursuits. Embrace the ups and downs as part of your unique journey, and find joy in the process of becoming the best version of yourself.

Maintaining a Healthy, Balanced Lifestyle for the Long Haul

Achieving your health and fitness goals is a significant accomplishment, but the real challenge lies in maintaining them over the long term. A healthy, balanced lifestyle isn't about short-term fixes or extreme measures; it's about sustainable habits that support your well-being in the long haul. By focusing on balance, consistency, and enjoyment, you can maintain your results while continuing to thrive physically and mentally.

What Does a Balanced Lifestyle Look Like?

A healthy, balanced lifestyle involves integrating habits that nourish your body and mind without feeling restrictive or overwhelming. Key components include:

1. **Nutritional Balance**
   Eating a variety of nutrient-dense foods that provide the vitamins, minerals, and energy your body needs. This includes lean proteins, whole grains, healthy fats, and plenty of fruits and vegetables.
2. **Regular Physical Activity**
   Engaging in a mix of cardio, strength training, and flexibility exercises to keep your body strong, agile, and energized.
3. **Mental Well-being**
   Prioritizing mental health through stress management, adequate sleep, and practices like mindfulness or meditation.
4. **Flexibility and Enjoyment**
   Allowing room for occasional indulgences and activities you love to ensure your lifestyle feels enjoyable and sustainable.

The Role of The Smoothie Diet in Long-Term Success

The Smoothie Diet is an excellent tool for maintaining a healthy lifestyle over the long term. Here's how it supports your goals:

1. **Convenience and Simplicity**
   Preparing smoothies is quick and easy, making it simple to stick to your nutrition plan even on busy days. This ensures you're consistently fueling your body with balanced meals.
2. **Nutrient-Dense and Satisfying**
   Smoothies are packed with essential nutrients, including fiber, protein, and healthy fats, which keep you full and energized throughout the day. They can also help curb cravings, making it easier to maintain your weight.
3. **Customizable and Versatile**
   Whether you're looking for a post-workout recovery drink, a quick breakfast, or a healthy snack, smoothies can be tailored to fit your needs and preferences. The variety helps prevent boredom and keeps your diet enjoyable.
4. **Sustainable for Long-Term Use**
   Unlike restrictive diets, The Smoothie Diet can be easily integrated into your routine as a long-term solution for balanced nutrition and weight maintenance.

Strategies for Long-Term Maintenance

1. **Set Realistic Expectations**
   Understand that weight maintenance doesn't mean your weight will stay the same every day. Minor fluctuations are normal. Focus on overall trends rather than daily changes.
2. **Keep Moving**
   Stay physically active by incorporating movement into your daily life. This could include regular workouts, walking, biking, or even taking the stairs instead of the elevator.

3. **Monitor Your Progress**

   Regularly check in with yourself through methods like tracking your meals, weighing yourself weekly, or noting how your clothes fit. This helps you stay on track without becoming overly fixated on numbers.

4. **Plan and Prep**

   Meal planning and preparation are key to maintaining a balanced diet. Keep your kitchen stocked with healthy staples, including smoothie ingredients, to avoid falling back on unhealthy choices during busy periods.

5. **Build a Support System**

   Surround yourself with people who encourage and support your healthy lifestyle. Share your journey with friends, join a fitness community, or find a workout buddy to keep each other accountable.

6. **Celebrate Milestones**

   Acknowledge and reward yourself for maintaining your healthy habits. Celebrating small victories reinforces positive behavior and keeps you motivated.

Managing Life's Challenges

Life is unpredictable, and there will be times when maintaining a healthy lifestyle feels more challenging. Here's how to navigate these periods:

1. **Be Flexible**

   Adapt your routine to fit your current circumstances. If you're traveling, find ways to stay active and make healthy food choices, such as packing protein-rich snacks or enjoying smoothies on the go.

2. **Learn from Setbacks**

   Treat setbacks as learning opportunities rather than failures. Reflect on what triggered the setback and how you can prevent it in the future.

3. **Focus on Small Wins**
   During tough times, focus on maintaining small, achievable habits like drinking enough water, preparing a healthy smoothie, or fitting in a 10-minute walk.

Long-Term Benefits of a Balanced Lifestyle

By maintaining a healthy, balanced lifestyle, you'll experience numerous benefits beyond weight maintenance:

- **Improved Energy Levels**
  Consistent nutrition and regular exercise keep your energy levels high, allowing you to enjoy daily activities with vitality.
- **Enhanced Mental Health**
  Healthy habits support mental well-being by reducing stress, improving sleep, and boosting mood.
- **Reduced Risk of Chronic Diseases**
  A balanced lifestyle lowers the risk of developing conditions like heart disease, diabetes, and hypertension.
- **Increased Longevity and Quality of Life**
  Healthy habits contribute to a longer, more active, and fulfilling life.

Final Thoughts

Transitioning from weight loss to maintenance mode is a rewarding phase that solidifies your hard-earned progress. Focus on consistency, mindfulness, and flexibility to enjoy lasting success and a balanced lifestyle.

Maintaining a healthy, balanced lifestyle is a lifelong commitment, but it doesn't have to be complicated or restrictive. Remember, consistency is more important than perfection, and every positive choice contributes to your long-term success. Embrace the journey and celebrate the small victories along the way, knowing that you're investing in a healthier, happier future.

Setbacks are inevitable, but they don't define your journey. Remember, consistency isn't about being perfect—it's about showing up, learning from setbacks, and continuing to move forward. Each step, no matter how small, brings you closer to your goals and helps you build a healthier, more sustainable lifestyle.

Conclusion:

Celebrating Your Transformation and Staying Fit & Fueled for Life

Congratulations on completing *Fit & Fueled: The Ultimate Guide to Nutrition and Exercise for Lasting Weight Loss*! This journey has been about more than shedding pounds; it's been about embracing a healthier, stronger, and more confident version of you. You've learned to fuel your body with nutritious choices, build a balanced fitness routine, and develop a resilient mindset that will carry you through life's challenges. Now, it's time to celebrate your transformation and focus on maintaining your progress for the long haul.

Celebrating Your Transformation
Your journey is a testament to your commitment, determination, and the power of small, consistent changes. Reflect on the progress you've made—not just in terms of physical changes, but also in your habits, mindset, and overall well-being. Celebrating your wins, no matter how small, reinforces your success and fuels your motivation to continue striving for your goals.

Think back to where you started and acknowledge how far you've come. Whether it's mastering meal prep, completing your first strength-training session, or finally breaking through a plateau, each step has brought you closer to a healthier, happier life.

Keep the Momentum Going: Resources for Continuous Growth
Sustaining your transformation is about more than maintenance; it's about continuous growth and evolution. Weight loss and fitness are lifelong commitments, and you have the tools to adapt to whatever challenges come your way. Here's how you can keep building on your success:

1. **Revisit Your Goals**

   As you progress, your goals may change. Reassess what you want to achieve—whether it's running a marathon, building muscle, or simply staying active—and adjust your plan accordingly.

2. **Leverage Support Systems**

   Surround yourself with a supportive community that shares your values. Whether it's joining a fitness group, following inspiring social media accounts, or enlisting a workout buddy, these connections can help keep you motivated.

3. **Explore New Challenges**

   Keep things exciting by trying new activities, recipes, or fitness routines. Variety not only prevents boredom but also challenges your body in different ways, promoting continued improvement.

4. **Rely on Trusted Resources**

   From revisiting the strategies outlined in this book to exploring additional tools like The Smoothie Diet for nutritious, convenient meals, staying informed and adaptable ensures you're always equipped for success.

Final Thoughts on Staying Fit & Fueled for Life

This guide has provided you with a comprehensive approach to lasting weight loss and lifelong health. From understanding nutrition basics to conquering weight-loss plateaus, you now have a roadmap to navigate the complexities of health and wellness. Remember, this journey isn't about perfection—it's about consistency, resilience, and enjoying the process.

Staying fit and fueled is a lifestyle, not a destination. By prioritizing your health, embracing challenges, and celebrating your wins, you're building a foundation for long-term success. The habits you've cultivated will not only help you maintain your progress but also empower you to thrive in every aspect of your life.

Call to Action

Your journey doesn't end here—it's only the beginning. Start by applying what you've learned today, and take the first step toward a lifetime of health and wellness. Share your progress, inspire others, and continue to explore resources that support your goals.

Ready to take your transformation even further? Stay connected with the *Fit & Fueled* community for tips, motivation, and updates to keep you inspired. Remember: every step forward, no matter how small, brings you closer to your best self.

Stay fit, stay fueled, and enjoy the life you've worked so hard to create!

Appendix

1. Nutrition Resources

Key Macronutrient Guidelines

- **Protein**: Essential for muscle repair and satiety. Aim for 1.2–2.0 grams per kilogram of body weight, depending on activity level.
- **Carbohydrates**: Primary energy source. Prioritize complex carbs like whole grains, vegetables, and fruits.
- **Fats**: Necessary for hormonal health and energy. Focus on unsaturated fats from nuts, seeds, and fish.

Superfoods for Weight Loss

- Leafy Greens: Spinach, kale, and arugula for nutrients and fiber.
- Lean Proteins: Chicken, fish, eggs, and plant-based proteins.
- High-Fiber Foods: Oats, chia seeds, and legumes to support digestion.

Meal Prep Tips

- Plan meals for the week ahead to stay on track.
- Use portion-controlled containers to prevent overeating.
- Rotate recipes to keep your meals exciting and flavorful.

2. Exercise References

Recommended Workouts

- **Cardio**:
    - Beginner: 20–30 minutes of brisk walking or cycling.
    - Intermediate: 30–45 minutes of jogging, swimming, or HIIT.
    - Advanced: Interval training with sprints or challenging terrains.
- **Strength Training**:
    - Beginner: Bodyweight exercises (squats, push-ups, planks).
    - Intermediate: Dumbbells or resistance bands for compound lifts.
    - Advanced: Free weights or gym machines with progressive overload.
- **Flexibility and Recovery**:
    - Daily stretching routines or yoga to improve mobility and prevent injury.

Weekly Workout Plan Example

Day	Activity	Focus
Monday	Cardio	Endurance
Tuesday	Strength Training	Upper Body
Wednesday	Yoga or Rest	Recovery
Thursday	Cardio (HIIT)	Fat Burn
Friday	Strength Training	Lower Body
Saturday	Outdoor Activity (Hiking)	Fun and Functional
Sunday	Rest or Active Recovery	Relaxation

3. Mindset and Habit Formation Tools

SMART Goal Setting

- **Specific**: Define exactly what you want to achieve (e.g., lose 10 pounds).
- **Measurable**: Use metrics to track progress (e.g., waist size, weight, or fitness level).
- **Achievable**: Ensure your goal is realistic within your timeline.
- **Relevant**: Align your goal with personal values and motivations.
- **Time-bound**: Set a deadline to maintain focus and urgency.

Motivation Strategies

- Identify your "why" to stay committed during challenges.
- Celebrate small wins to maintain momentum.
- Surround yourself with a supportive community.

4. Supplemental Tools

The Smoothie Diet for Weight Loss and Maintenance
Smoothies can be a practical and delicious way to fuel your body while supporting weight loss.

- **Sample Recipe:**
    - 1 cup unsweetened almond milk
    - 1 scoop protein powder
    - 1 cup spinach
    - ½ banana
    - 1 tablespoon chia seeds
    - Blend until smooth for a nutrient-packed snack or meal replacement.

Tracking Progress

- **Measurements**: Take circumference measurements of key areas (waist, hips, thighs).
- **Photos**: Document your journey with progress photos.
- **Journals**: Log workouts, meals, and reflections to identify patterns and celebrate achievements.

---

5. Additional Resources

Recommended Apps

- **MyFitnessPal**: For tracking meals and calories.
- **Strava**: For tracking cardio workouts.
- **Headspace**: For mindfulness and stress management.

Further Reading

- *The New Rules of Lifting* by Lou Schuler
- *The Complete Guide to Nutrition* by Anita Bean
- *Atomic Habits* by James Clear

Online Communities

- Reddit: r/Fitness and r/LoseIt for advice and support.
- Facebook Groups: Look for local or global fitness communities.

---

6. Contact and Acknowledgments

Feedback

Your journey is unique, and I'd love to hear about your progress and experiences. Feel free to share your success stories or ask questions by reaching out to [Your Contact Information].

Thank You

Thank you for trusting *Fit & Fueled* as your guide. This book was written to empower and inspire you to achieve your best self. I'm honored to be part of your journey.

References

The following resources were consulted to provide evidence-based, accurate, and practical information for *Fit & Fueled: The Ultimate Guide to Nutrition and Exercise for Lasting Weight Loss*. These references ensure the credibility and reliability of the content presented in this book.

Nutrition References

1. Academy of Nutrition and Dietetics. (2021). *Dietary Guidelines for Americans, 2020-2025*. U.S. Department of Agriculture and U.S. Department of Health and Human Services.
   - https://www.dietaryguidelines.gov
2. Harvard T.H. Chan School of Public Health. (n.d.). *Healthy Eating Plate*.
   - https://www.hsph.harvard.edu/nutritionsource/healthy-eating-plate
3. Mayo Clinic Staff. (2023). *Dietary fiber: Essential for a healthy diet*. Mayo Clinic.
   - https://www.mayoclinic.org
4. National Institutes of Health. (2022). *Understanding Macronutrients: Protein, Carbohydrates, and Fats*.
   - https://www.nih.gov
5. Precision Nutrition. (2021). *The Essentials of Nutrition and Coaching*.

Exercise References

1. American Council on Exercise (ACE). (2023). *The Benefits of Strength Training for Weight Loss.*
   o https://www.acefitness.org
2. American Heart Association. (2022). *Recommendations for Physical Activity in Adults.*
   o https://www.heart.org
3. Schoenfeld, B. J. (2010). *The Mechanisms of Muscle Hypertrophy and Their Application to Resistance Training.* Journal of Strength and Conditioning Research.
   o DOI: 10.1519/JSC.0b013e3181e840f3
4. Tabata, I., et al. (1996). *Effects of Moderate-Intensity Endurance and High-Intensity Intermittent Training on Anaerobic Capacity and VO2 Max.* Medicine & Science in Sports & Exercise.
   o DOI: 10.1249/00005768-199610000-00018
5. World Health Organization. (2020). *Global Recommendations on Physical Activity for Health.*
   o https://www.who.int

Behavior and Mindset References

1. Clear, J. (2018). *Atomic Habits: An Easy & Proven Way to Build Good Habits & Break Bad Ones.* Avery Publishing.
2. Duhigg, C. (2014). *The Power of Habit: Why We Do What We Do in Life and Business.* Random House Trade Paperbacks.
3. Ryan, R. M., & Deci, E. L. (2000). *Self-Determination Theory and the Facilitation of Intrinsic Motivation, Social Development, and Well-Being.* American Psychologist.
   o DOI: 10.1037/0003-066X.55.1.68
4. Wood, W., & Neal, D. T. (2007). *A New Look at Habits and the Habit-Goal Interface.* Psychological Review.
   o DOI: 10.1037/0033-295X.114.4.843

<u>**Supplemental Resources**</u>

1. USDA Food Composition Databases. (n.d.).
   - https://fdc.nal.usda.gov
2. National Sleep Foundation. (2022). *Sleep and Weight Loss: Understanding the Connection.*
   - https://www.sleepfoundation.org
3. Centers for Disease Control and Prevention (CDC). (2023). *Healthy Weight, Nutrition, and Physical Activity.*
   - https://www.cdc.gov
4. Headspace. (n.d.). *Guided Meditation for Stress and Motivation.*
   - https://www.headspace.com
5. The Smoothie Diet by Drew S. (n.d.). *21-Day Program for Weight Loss and Maintenance.*

Disclosure

This e-book, *Fit & Fueled: The Ultimate Guide to Nutrition and Exercise for Lasting Weight Loss*, is fully AI-generated. It has been created using advanced artificial intelligence technology to provide insights, tips, and strategies on nutrition, exercise, and sustainable weight loss. While every effort has been made to ensure accuracy and reliability, it is important to note that this book should not replace professional medical or fitness advice.

Readers are encouraged to consult with healthcare providers, certified nutritionists, or fitness professionals before making significant changes to their diet or exercise routines. The information in this book is intended for general educational and informational purposes only.

Thank you for choosing this guide, and we hope it helps you on your journey toward a healthier, fitter, and more fueled lifestyle!

www.ingramcontent.com/pod-product-compliance
Lightning Source LLC
Chambersburg PA
CBHW061633250726
48659CB00004B/1191